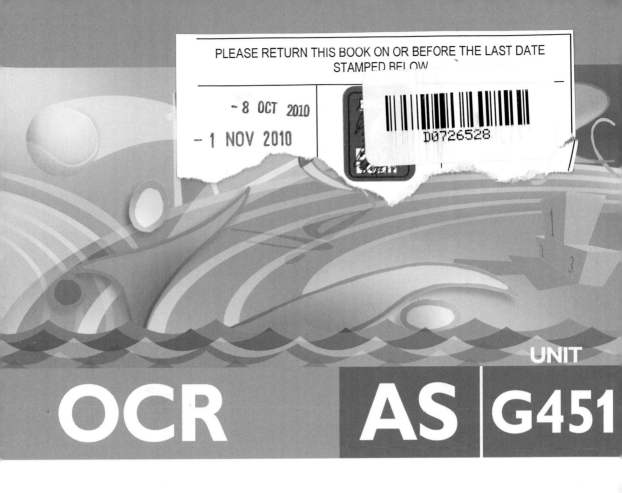

UNIT

OCR   AS G451

Physical Education

An Introduction to Physical Education

Symond Burrows, Micha
and Sue Young

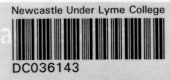

Philip Allan Updates, an imprint of Hodder Education, part of Hachette UK, Market Place, Deddington, Oxfordshire OX15 0SE

Orders

Bookpoint Ltd, 130 Milton Park, Abingdon, Oxfordshire, OX14 4SB
tel: 01235 827720
fax: 01235 400454
e-mail: uk.orders@bookpoint.co.uk
Lines are open 9.00 a.m.–5.00 p.m., Monday to Saturday, with a 24-hour message answering service. You can also order through the Philip Allan Updates website: www.philipallan.co.uk

© Philip Allan Updates 2009

ISBN 978-0-340-94789-0
First printed 2009
Impression number   5   4   3   2   1
Year   2014   2013   2012   2011   2010   2009

This Guide has been written specifically to support students preparing for the OCR AS Physical Education Unit G451 examination. The content has been neither approved nor endorsed by OCR and remains the sole responsibility of the authors.

Printed by MPG Books, Bodmin

Hachette UK's policy is to use papers that are natural, renewable and recyclable products and made from wood grown in sustainable forests. The logging and manufacturing processes are expected to conform to the environmental regulations of the country of origin.

P01313

Contents

Introduction

■ ■ ■

Content Guidance

■ ■ ■

introduction

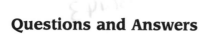

Questions and Answers

Introduction

About this guide

This unit guide is written to help you prepare for **Unit G451: An Introduction to Physical Education**. There are three sections to this guide:

- **Introduction** — this provides advice on how to use the unit guide, an explanation of the skills required for Unit G451 and suggestions for effective revision.
- **Content Guidance** — this summarises the specification content of Unit G451.
- **Questions and Answers** — this provides examples of questions from various topic areas, together with student answers and examiner's comments on how these could have been improved.

The specification

In order to make a good start to Unit G451, it is important to have a close look at the specification. If you do not have a copy of this, either ask your teacher for one or download it from the OCR website, **www.ocr.org.uk**.

In addition to describing the content of the unit (which sometimes provides detail that could earn you marks), the specification gives information about the unit tests. The specification also provides information about other skills required in Unit G451. For example, using the knowledge and understanding gained as a basis for improving the effectiveness and efficiency of your performance in roles such as performer, leader or coach and official. The application of knowledge will enable you to evaluate lifestyle choices in relation to their impact on body systems and lifelong participation in physical activity.

You also need to develop the skills of interpreting and drawing graphs and diagrams.

Study skills and revision strategies

All students need good study skills to be successful. This section provides advice and guidance on how to study AS physical education, together with some strategies for effective revision.

Organising your notes

PE students often accumulate a large quantity of notes, so it is useful to keep this information in an organised manner. The presentation is important; good notes should be clear and concise. You could try organising your notes under main headings and subheadings, with key points highlighted using capitals, italics or colour. Numbered lists can be useful, as can the presentation of information in table form and simple diagrams. For example:

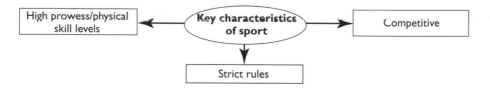

It is a good idea to file your notes in specification order, using a consistent series of headings, as illustrated below:

Unit G451, Section B: acquiring movement skills
Classification of motor skills Position and justify examples of movement skills on the following continua: • muscular involvement (gross–fine) • environmental influence (open–closed) • continuity (discrete–serial–continuous) • pacing (externally paced–self paced) • difficulty (simple–complex) • organisation (high–low)

At a convenient time after lessons, check your understanding of your notes. If anything is still unclear, you could ask a friend to explain, do some further reading, or ask your teacher for help.

Organising your time

It is a good idea to make a revision timetable to ensure you use your time effectively. This should allow enough time to cover all the relevant material. However, it must also be realistic. For many students, revising for longer than an hour at a time becomes counterproductive, so allow time for short relaxation breaks or exercise to refresh the body and mind.

Revision strategies

To revise a topic effectively, you should work carefully through your notes, using a copy of the specification to make sure everything is covered. Summarise your notes on the key points using the tips offered above. Topic cue cards, with a summary of key facts and visual representations of the material can be useful. These are easily carried around for quick revision.

In many ways you should prepare for a unit test like an athlete prepares for a major event, such as the Olympic Games. An athlete trains every day for weeks or months before the event, practising the required skills in order to achieve the best result on the day. So it is with exam preparation: everything you do should contribute to your chances of success in the unit test.

The following points summarise some of the strategies that you may wish to use to make sure your revision is as effective as possible:
- Use a revision timetable.
- Ideally, spend time revising in a quiet room, sitting upright at a desk or table, with no distractions (turn your television and mobile phone off).
- Test yourself regularly to assess the effectiveness of your revision. Ask yourself: 'Which techniques work best?' 'What are the gaps in my knowledge?' Remember to revise what you *don't* know.
- Practise past paper questions to highlight gaps in your knowledge and to improve your exam technique. You will also become familiar with the terminology used in exam questions.
- Spend some time doing 'active revision', such as:
  - discussing topics with fellow students or teachers
  - summarising your notes
  - compiling revision cue cards
  - answering previous test questions and self-checking against mark schemes

Revision progress

Preparation for exams is a personal thing — you should do what works best for you. You could also draw up, and use, a 'revision progress' table for each topic. An example is shown below.

Complete column 2 to show how you have progressed with your revision:
- N = not revised yet
- P = partly revised
- F = fully revised

Complete column 3 to show how confident you are with the topic:
- 5 = high degree of confidence
- 1 = minimal confidence — the practice questions were poorly answered

The table should be updated as your revision progresses.

Section A Anatomy and physiology

The skeletal and muscular systems

Topic	Revised (N/P/F)	Self-evaluation (1–5)
Joints: movement, muscles		
The role of muscular contraction		
Movement analysis of physical activity		
Muscle fibre types in relation to choice of physical activity		
Warm-up/cool-down		
Impact of different types of physical activity on the skeletal and muscular systems		

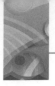
The unit test

The Unit G451 test is divided into three sections:
- Section A — Anatomy and Physiology
- Section B — Acquiring Movement Skills
- Section C — Socio-cultural Studies Relating to Participation in Physical Activity

The test comprises three compulsory structured questions — one from each section, each worth 30 marks. Each question is broken into parts. Mark allocations vary, but most parts are worth 2–5 marks. The final part of each question is worth 10 marks, which includes an assessment of the quality of your written communication. There are 90 marks available in this test, which count for 60% of the total AS GCE PE marks. You will have 2 hours to complete the test.

Write clearly in the spaces provided in the answer booklet. Avoid writing anything that you want to be marked in the margins because it might not be seen by the examiner if the paper is scanned for online marking. If you need more room for your answer, look for space at the bottom of the page or use the spare sheets at the end of the booklet. If you do this, alert the examiner by adding 'continued below', or 'continued on page X'.

Some words may be emphasised (in bold type). This is to draw your attention to key words or phrases that you need to consider in order to answer the question.

There are a number of terms commonly used in unit tests. It is important that you understand the meaning of each of these terms and that you answer the question appropriately.
- **Analyse/critically evaluate/discuss** — put both sides of an argument, stating your opinions as appropriate.
- **Apply/demonstrate your knowledge** — use practical sporting examples to illustrate your understanding of theoretical content.
- **Compare** — point out similarities and differences.
- **Define** — give a clear, concise statement outlining what is meant by a particular term.
- **Describe** — provide an accurate account of the main points in relation to the task set.
- **Explain** — give reasons to justify statements and opinions given in your answer.
- **State/give/list/identify** — give a concise, factual answer.

Whatever the question style, you must read the wording carefully, underline or highlight key words or phrases, think about your response and allocate time according to the number of marks available. Further advice and guidance on answering Unit G451 questions is provided in the Questions and Answers section of this guide.

Content
Guidance

Unit G451 comprises three sections. Section A is called **Anatomy and Physiology**, Section B is **Acquiring Movement Skills**, and Section C is **Sociocultural Studies Relating to Participation in Physical Activity**.

Section A is concerned with the impact of physical activity on the body systems and on a young individual's participation and performance in physical activity, as part of a balanced, active and healthy lifestyle.

Section B relates to the acquisition of movement skills that impact on a young person's participation and performance in physical activity, as part of a balanced, active and healthy lifestyle.

Section C focuses on the importance of physical activity in modern-day society. It aims to develop knowledge and understanding of a range of sociocultural factors that influence regular participation and the achievement of sporting excellence.

This Content Guidance section summarises the key information that you need to understand and apply in the G451 unit test. It also includes useful examiner's tips and hints on 'What the examiner will expect you to be able to do'.

Remember that this Content Guidance is designed to support your revision and should be used in conjunction with your textbook, your own revision notes and other resources.

Anatomy and physiology

The skeletal and muscular systems

Joints

The skeleton is a framework held together by joints. Joints are necessary for muscles to lever bones, thus creating movement. A joint is formed where two or more bones meet. Joints are classified by how much movement they allow. There are three types:

- **fibrous** joints allow no movement and the bones are held together by fibrous, connective tissue, e.g. the cranium
- **cartilaginous** joints allow slight movement and the bones are separated by cartilage, e.g. the vertebrae
- **synovial** joints allow movement in one or more directions

Synovial joints

Synovial joints are the most common type of joint. They have a fluid-filled cavity surrounded by an articular capsule. Hyaline or articular cartilage occurs where the bones come into contact with each other. There are six types of synovial joint:

- ball-and-socket joint — hip and shoulder
- hinge joint — ankle, knee and elbow
- pivot joint — radio-ulna and between the axis and atlas in the neck
- saddle joint — thumb
- condyloid joint — wrist
- gliding joint — between vertebrae in the spine

Movement terminology

There are a number of technical terms that you should be familiar with:

- **flexion** — a decrease in the angle that occurs around a joint
- **extension** — an increase in the angle that occurs around a joint
- **horizontal flexion** — lifting the arm up and across the body
- **horizontal extension** — lowering the arm down and across the body
- **abduction** — movement occurring away from the midline of the body
- **adduction** — movement occurring towards the midline of the body
- **rotation** — movement of a bone around its axis, which can be inward (medial) or outward (lateral)
- **circumduction** — the lower end of the bone moves around in a circle, e.g. on rotating the shoulder, circumduction occurs in the bones of the wrist
- **lateral flexion** — bending sideways
- **plantar flexion** — bending the foot downwards away from the tibia (standing on your tiptoes)
- **palmar flexion** — bending the hand downwards towards the inside of the forearm

- **dorsiflexion** — bending the foot upwards towards the tibia or bending the hand backwards
- **pronation** — facing the palm of the hand downwards
- **supination** — facing the palm of the hand upwards (carrying a 'soup' bowl may help you to remember!)

Synovial joints, movement and agonist muscles

These are summarised in the tables below.

Ball-and-socket joints

Joint	Articulating bones	Movement	Agonist
Hip	Acetabulum of the pelvis and femur	Flexion	Iliopsoas
		Extension	Gluteus maximus
		Lateral (outward) rotation	Gluteus maximus
		Medial (inward) rotation	Gluteus minimus
		Abduction	Gluteus medius
		Adduction	Adductors (longus, brevis and magnus)
Shoulder	Glenoid fossa of the scapula and humerus	Flexion	Anterior deltoid
		Extension	Posterior deltoid
		Lateral (outward) rotation	Infraspinatus
		Medial (inward) rotation	Subscapularis
		Abduction	Middle deltoid
		Adduction	Pectoralis major
		Horizontal flexion	Pectoralis major
		Horizontal extension	Trapezius

Hinge joints

Joint	Articulating bones	Movement	Agonist
Elbow	Radius, ulna and humerus	Flexion	Biceps brachii
		Extension	Triceps brachii
Knee	Tibia and femur	Flexion	Biceps femoris
		Extension	Rectus femoris
Ankle	Tibia, fibula and talus	Plantarflexion	Gastrocnemius
		Dorsiflexion	Tibialis anterior

Pivot joint

Joint	Articulating bones	Movement	Agonist
Radio-ulnar	Radius and ulna	Pronation	Pronator teres
		Supination	Supinator

Gliding joint

Joint	Articulating bones	Movement	Agonist
Spine	Vertebral arches	Flexion	Rectus abdominus
		Extension	Erector spinae group
		Lateral flexion	External obliques
		Rotation (to the opposite side)	Internal obliques

Condyloid joint

Joint	Articulating bones	Movement	Agonist
Wrist	Carpals, radius, ulna	Palmarflexion	Wrist flexors
		Dorsiflexion	Wrist extensors

Types of muscular contraction

A muscle can contract in three different ways, depending on the muscle action that is required.

Concentric contraction

The muscle shortens under tension. For example, during the upward phase of an arm curl, the biceps brachii performs a concentric contraction as it shortens to produce flexion of the elbow.

Eccentric contraction

The muscle lengthens under tension (and does not relax). When a muscle contracts eccentrically it is acting as a brake to help control the movement of the body part during negative work (e.g. landing from a standing jump). Here the quadriceps muscles are performing negative work as they are supporting the weight of the body during landing. The knee joint is in the flexed position but the quadriceps muscles are unable to relax as the weight of the body ensures that they lengthen under tension.

Isometric contraction

The muscle contracts without lengthening or shortening. The result is that no movement occurs. An isometric contraction occurs when a muscle acts as a fixator or against a resistance.

Functions of skeletal muscle

A muscle can perform three functions:
- **agonist** — the muscle shortens under tension to produce movement

- **antagonist** — the muscle relaxes or lengthens to allow the agonist to shorten
- **fixator** — the muscle increases in tension but no movement occurs. A fixator is normally located at the joint where the origin of the agonist occurs. For example, in the upward phase of an arm curl, the biceps brachii contracts and is the agonist. Its origin is on the shoulder, so the deltoid acts as a fixator during this movement.

Muscle structure

There are three main types of muscle fibre:
- type I — **slow oxidative** (slow twitch)
- type IIa — **fast oxidative glycolytic** (fast twitch)
- type IIb — **fast glycolytic** (fast twitch)

Skeletal muscles contain a mixture of all three types of fibre but not in equal proportions. The mix is mainly genetically determined. The fibres are grouped into motor units and only one type of fibre occurs in any particular unit.

The relative proportion of each fibre type varies in the same muscles of different people. For example, elite endurance athletes have a greater proportion of slow-twitch fibres in their leg muscles while elite sprinters have a greater proportion of fast-twitch fibres. Postural muscles tend to have a greater proportion of slow-twitch fibres as they are involved in maintaining body position over long periods of time.

All three types of fibre have specific characteristics that allow them to perform their role successfully. These are summarised in the tables below.

Structural characteristic	Type I	Type IIa	Type IIb
Size	Small	Medium	Large
Glycogen store	Low	Medium	High
Capillaries	Many	Many	Few
Mitochondria	Many	Many	Few
Myoglobin concentration	High	High	Low

Functional characteristic	Type I	Type IIa	Type IIb
Contraction speed	Slow	Fast	Fast
Force produced	Low	Medium	High
Aerobic capacity	High	Medium	Low
Anaerobic capacity	Low	High	High
Tendency to fatigue	Low	Medium	High

Physiological effects of warming up and cooling down

A warm-up has the following physiological effects:
- The release of adrenaline increases heart rate and dilates the capillaries. The vasomotor centre ensures that vasodilation occurs, so that more blood flows (due

to the increase in cardiac output) to the working muscles. These responses allow more oxygen to be delivered to the skeletal muscles.

- Muscle temperature increases, which enables oxygen to dissociate more easily from haemoglobin and increases enzyme activity, making energy readily available.
- An increase in the speed of nerve impulse conduction increases alertness.
- The increase in muscle temperature leads to an increase in elasticity of the muscle fibres, which increases the speed and force of muscle contraction.
- An increased production of synovial fluid leads to efficient movement at joints.
- A reduction in muscle viscosity improves the coordination between antagonistic pairs, which increases the speed and strength of contraction.
- The increase in enzyme activity in the warmer muscle fibres increases the speed and strength of muscle contraction.

A cool-down at the end of any physical activity helps to return the body to its pre-exercise state more quickly. It consists of some form of light exercise to keep the heart rate elevated. This keeps blood flow high and allows oxygen to be flushed through the muscles, removing and oxidising any lactic acid that remains. Performing light exercise also allows the skeletal muscle pump to keep working, preventing blood from pooling in the veins. Light exercise should be followed by some static stretches.

Impact of exercise on the skeletal and muscular systems

Low-impact aerobic activities

Osteoporosis (weakening of the bone) is caused by the loss of calcium salts in a process called demineralisation. Taking part in low-impact aerobic activities can reverse this trend. The bones become stronger due to increased calcium deposits and the strength of muscles, tendons and ligaments increases. Low-impact activity also avoids over-use injuries by varying the line of stress on bones.

Osteoarthritis is a deterioration of the joint cartilage and the development of bony spurs on the bones at the edge of the joints. It usually affects the knees, hips, hands, feet and spine. Low-impact aerobic activities can help mild osteoarthritis by increasing blood flow, thus nourishing cartilage and bone and strengthening the joints, causing them to be more stable.

Strength training and core stability

This type of training can cause hypertrophy of the muscles. The increase in muscle strength leads to an increase in joint stability. For example, core stability exercises can increase the strength of the rotator cuff muscles, which increases stability in the shoulder joint as well as reducing the likelihood of problems with the lumbar vertebrae. Increasing the strength in the quadriceps muscles helps to stabilise tracking and knee function. Strengthening exercises can also help with mild osteoarthritis by decreasing joint stiffness and strengthening the muscles around a joint, to give protection and absorb shock.

However, strength training involves a lot of eccentric muscle contractions, which can cause muscle damage. For example, in a squat, the quadriceps muscles contract concentrically during the upward phase to straighten the knee but eccentrically during the downward (bending) phase. This means that the muscles cannot relax throughout the squat. Overdoing the number of squats can cause muscle damage.

High-impact activities

High-impact activities involve contact, which can cause damage to the growth plate. This is the softer part of young people's bones where growth occurs. Growth plates are found at the ends of bones and are the weakest sections of the skeleton. They are susceptible to injury. Immediate treatment is required in the event of injury as it can affect how the bone may grow.

Medial or cruciate ligament damage in the knee can result from side impact. Heavy impact to the shoulder joint can cause dislocation due to the shallow joint cavity.

Flexibility training

Flexibility training involves stretching muscles and connective tissue. Regular and repeated stretching can elongate the soft tissue, which may be beneficial in avoiding injury. Tendons, ligaments and particularly muscle tissue surrounding a joint increase their resting length due to greater elasticity. This increases the range of movement around the joint. However, extreme flexibility can stretch ligaments and lead to a lack of stability.

Activities involving repetitive movements or over-use

Repetitive stress injuries occur when too much stress is placed on part of the body. The result is inflammation of the bursa, wearing down of the articular/hyaline cartilage in joints and muscle strain or tissue damage. Over-use injuries in children and teenagers usually occur at the growth plates. The most common repetitive stress injuries occur at the elbows, shoulders, knees and heels.

Speed and agility training

This allows muscles to retain more elasticity/elastin, which means they can contract with more speed and power.

What the examiner will expect you to be able to do

- Apply knowledge of movement to physical activity, for example analyse all the movement at the joints for a particular skill. Learning the movement analysis tables will give you all the necessary information.
- Identify activities where each muscle fibre type is predominant and identify the structural and functional characteristics of specific fibre types.
- Analyse the effects of a warm-up and cool-down in relation to quality of performance.
- Critically evaluate the impact of different types of physical activity on the skeletal and muscular systems.

Motion and movement

Newton's laws of motion

Newton's first law (law of inertia)
A body continues in its state of rest or uniform motion in a straight line, unless compelled to change that state by external forces exerted upon it.

For example, a ball (the body) will remain on the penalty spot (in a state of rest) until a player kicks it (an external force is exerted upon it).

Newton's second law (law of acceleration)
The rate of change in momentum of a body (or the acceleration for a body of constant mass) is proportional to the applied force, and the change takes place in the direction in which the force acts.

For example, when a player kicks (force applied) the ball during the game, the acceleration of the ball (rate of change of momentum) is proportional to the size of the force. So, the harder the ball is kicked the further and faster it will go.

Newton's third law (law of reaction)
To every action there is an equal and opposite reaction.

For example, when a footballer jumps up (action) to win a header, a force is exerted on the ground in order to gain height. At the same time, the ground exerts an upward force (equal and opposite reaction) on the player.

Motion

Motion can be:
- **linear** — motion in a straight or curved line, as long as all parts move the same distance in the same direction and at the same speed (e.g. tobogganing in a straight line, or the curved flight of a shot put)
- **angular** — movement around a fixed point or axis (e.g. a somersault)
- **general** — a combination of linear and angular motion (e.g. in the javelin throw, the body moves in a straight line on the approach but the arm moves in a circular motion during the throwing action)

Force

A force can be described as a 'push' or a 'pull'. It can cause a body at rest to move, or cause a moving body to stop, slow down, speed up or change direction. A force can be measured in terms of:
- size or magnitude — this depends on the size and number of muscle fibres used
- direction — if a force is applied through the middle of an object, it will move in the same direction as the force
- the position of application — applying a force straight through the centre results in movement in a straight line (linear motion); applying a force off-centre results in spin (angular motion)

Centre of mass

The centre of mass is the point of balance. For someone in a standing position, the centre of mass is in the hip region. A balanced stable position depends on:

- the centre of mass being over the base of support
- the line of gravity running through the middle of the base of support
- the number of contact points — the more contact points, the more stable the position (e.g. a headstand has more contact points than a handstand, so is a more stable position)
- the mass of the performer — the greater the mass, the more stability there is

What the examiner will expect you to be able to do
- Relate each of Newton's laws of motion to a practical example.
- Understand the effects of size, direction and application of force, and apply to sporting examples.
- Name a balance and describe the factors that affect its performance — handstand and headstand are the easiest.

Response of the heart to physical activity

The conduction system

Blood flows through the heart in a controlled manner, in through the atria and out through the ventricles. Heart muscle is described as **myogenic** because the beat starts in the heart muscle itself, with an electrical impulse in the **sinoatrial node** (SA node or pacemaker). This electrical impulse then spreads through the heart in what is often described as a wave of excitation (analogous to a Mexican wave).

From the SA node, the electrical impulse spreads through the walls of the atria, causing them to contract and forcing blood into the ventricles. The impulse then passes through the **atrioventricular node** (AV node) located in the atrioventricular septum and down through specialised fibres called the **bundle of His**. This is located in the septum separating the two ventricles. The bundle of His branches into two bundle branches and then into smaller bundles called Purkyne fibres, which spread throughout the ventricles, causing them to contract.

The cardiac cycle

The cardiac cycle describes the emptying and filling of the heart. It involves a number of stages:

- Diastole phase — the chambers relax and fill with blood.
- Systole phase — the heart contracts and forces blood either round the heart or out of the heart to the lungs and the body.

Each complete cardiac cycle takes approximately 0.8 seconds. The diastole phase takes about 0.5 seconds, the systole phase 0.3 seconds. The cardiac cycle is summarised in the table below:

Stage	Action	Result
Atrial systole	Atrial walls contract	Blood is forced through the bicuspid and tricuspid valves into the ventricles.
Atrial diastole	Atrial walls relax	Blood enters the right atrium via the vena cava and the left atrium via the pulmonary vein but cannot pass into the ventricles because the tricuspid and bicuspid valves are closed.
Ventricular systole	Venticular walls contract	Pressure of blood opens the semilunar valves and blood is ejected into the pulmonary artery to the lungs and into the aorta to the body. The tricuspid and bicuspid valves close.
Ventricular diastole	Ventricular walls relax	Blood enters from the atria (passive ventricular filling, not due to atrial contraction). The semilunar valves close.

Linking the conduction system and the cardiac cycle

The cardiac cycle describes the flow of blood through the heart during one heartbeat. Because the heart generates its own electrical impulses, this flow of blood is controlled by the conduction system.

- The impulse initiates at the SA node and travels across the atria, causing them to contract.
- The AV node receives the impulse and conducts it down the bundle of His, the bundle branches and the Purkyne fibres.
- The ventricles then contract.

Cardiac terms

Stroke volume is the amount of blood pumped out by the left ventricle in each contraction. The average resting stroke volume is approximately 70 ml. Stroke volume can be determined by the following:

- Venous return — the volume of blood returning to the heart via the veins. If venous return increases, stroke volume also increases (if more blood enters the heart then more blood is pumped out).
- The elasticity of the cardiac fibres — the more the cardiac fibres stretch during the diastole phase of the cardiac cycle, the greater the force of contraction. A greater force of contraction can increase stroke volume. This is **Starling's law**.
- The contractility of the cardiac tissue (myocardium) — the greater the contractility of the cardiac tissue, the greater the force of contraction. This results in an increase in stroke volume.

Heart rate is the number of times the heart beats per minute. The average resting heart rate is around 72 beats per minute.

Cardiac output is the amount of blood pumped out by the left ventricle per minute. It is equal to stroke volume multiplied by heart rate.

cardiac output (Q) = stroke volume × heart rate

$Q = 70 \times 72$

$Q = 5040\,ml$ (5.04 litres)

Heart rate response to exercise

Heart rate increases with exercise until it reaches a maximum, but how much it increases depends on the intensity of the exercise. The graphs below illustrate the changes in heart rate during maximal exercise such as sprinting and submaximal exercise such as jogging.

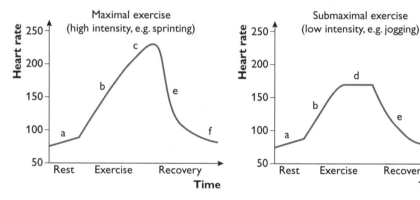

Key to the graphs:

a = the **anticipatory rise** due to the action of the hormone adrenaline, which stimulates the SA node to increase heart rate

b = a sharp rise in heart rate at the beginning of exercise, due mainly to anaerobic work

c = the heart rate continuing to rise due to maximal workloads stressing the anaerobic systems

d = a steady state as the athlete is able to meet the oxygen demand required for the activity (reaching a plateau)

e = a rapid decline in heart rate as soon as the exercise stops, because there is a decrease in the demand for oxygen by the working muscles

f = a slow recovery as the body systems return to resting levels (but the heart rate remains elevated to rid the body of waste products such as lactic acid)

Maximum heart rate can be approximated by subtracting the performer's age from 220.

Cardiac output response to exercise

Regular aerobic training results in hypertrophy of the cardiac muscle, i.e. the heart gets bigger. This affects stroke volume and heart rate, and therefore cardiac output.

A bigger heart pumps out more blood per beat (increased stroke volume). In other words, the end diastolic volume of the ventricle increases. If the ventricle can contract with more force and push out more blood, the heart does not have to beat so often. Therefore the resting heart rate decreases. This is called **bradycardia**. The increase in stroke volume and decrease in resting heart rate mean that cardiac output at rest remains unchanged. However, during exercise, an increase in heart rate, coupled with the increase in stroke volume, results in an increase in cardiac output. Cardiac output increases as the intensity of exercise increases until maximum exercise capacity is achieved and a plateau is reached.

The following table shows the differences in cardiac output (to the nearest litre) in a trained and an untrained individual at rest and during exercise. The individuals are aged 18, so their maximum heart rate is 202 beats per minute (bpm).

Individual	Condition	SV/ml	HR/bpm	Q/litres
Untrained	Rest	70	72	5
	Exercise	120	202	24
Trained	Rest	85	60	5
	Exercise	170	202	34

This increase in cardiac output has huge benefits for trained individuals. It means that more blood, and therefore more oxygen, is transported to the working muscles. In addition, when the body starts to exercise, the distribution of blood flow changes — a higher proportion of blood passes to the working muscles and less goes to other organs.

Stroke volume response to exercise

Stroke volume increases as exercise intensity increases but only up to 40–60% of maximum effort. Once a performer reaches this point, stroke volume levels out. One explanation is that the increased heart rate near maximum effort results in a shorter diastolic phase. The ventricles have less time to fill up with blood, so they cannot pump as much out.

Control of heart rate

Neural control

The autonomic nervous system comprises the **sympathetic system** and the **parasympathetic system**. The sympathetic system stimulates the heart to beat faster; the parasympathetic system returns the heart to its resting level. The **cardiac control centre** located in the medulla oblongata of the brain coordinates the two systems. The cardiac control centre is stimulated by:

- chemoreceptors (which detect chemical changes, e.g. carbon dioxide, lactic acid, oxygen)
- baroreceptors (which detect changes in blood pressure)
- proprioceptors (which detect movement)

This centre then sends an impulse through either the sympathetic or parasympathetic system to the sinoatrial node of the heart.

Hormonal control

Adrenaline and noradrenaline are stress hormones that are released by the adrenal glands. Exercise causes a stress-induced adrenaline response, which results in the following:

- stimulation of the SA node (pacemaker), which results in an increase in both the speed and force of heart muscle contraction
- an increase in blood pressure due to constriction of blood vessels
- an increase in blood glucose levels — glucose is used by the muscles for energy

Intrinsic control

During exercise, the heart becomes warmer, so heart rate increases. (A drop in temperature results in a reduced heart rate.) In addition, venous return increases, which stretches the cardiac muscle, stimulating the SA node. This, in turn, increases heart rate and the force of contraction of the heart muscle. As a result, stroke volume increases.

Effects of training on the heart

Physical activity causes the following changes to the heart:

- **Athlete's heart** is the common term for an enlarged heart caused by repeated strenuous aerobic exercise. The chambers of the heart become enlarged, which allows them to fill with more blood during diastole. Hence more blood can be pumped out per beat, so the heart has to contract less frequently.
- **Hypertrophy** of the myocardium means that the heart muscle gets bigger and stronger. This results in bradycardia and an increase in stroke volume.
- Maximum cardiac output increases but cardiac output at rest and during submaximal exercise remains the same.
- Increased capillarisation of the heart muscle increases the efficiency of oxygen diffusion into the myocardium.
- Increased contractility — resistance or strength training causes an increase in the force of heart contractions due to a thickening of the ventricular myocardium. This increases stroke volume and ejection fraction.

Lack of physical activity is one of the major risk factors associated with heart disease. Exercise helps the heart to become stronger, enabling it to pump more blood around the body.

Heart conditions related to a lack of exercise include the following:

- **Coronary heart disease**. Studies show that regular physical activity, coupled with a diet low in high-fat foods, is the best way to prevent heart disease. Medical experts recommend 30 minutes of physical activity five times per week. Moderate aerobic exercise can reduce cholesterol and lipid levels, including low-density lipoprotein (LDL — the bad cholesterol). Aerobic exercise can also increase levels of high-density lipoprotein (HDL — the good cholesterol), which is associated with a decrease in coronary heart disease. Resistance training has been shown to lower heart rate and blood pressure after exercise. This will reduce the risk of heart disease.

- A **heart attack** occurs when part of the heart muscle dies because it has been starved of oxygen as a result of coronary heart disease. Regular aerobic exercise, such as brisk walking, jogging, swimming and cycling, can help to prevent a heart attack.
- **Angina** is a symptom of coronary heart disease. It manifests as chest pain when the muscles do not receive enough blood. Exercises that train and strengthen the chest muscles will help to protect against angina.

What the examiner will expect you to be able to do
- Describe the link between the conduction system and the cardiac cycle.
- Explain the changes in heart rate, cardiac output and stroke volume during different intensities of physical activity. Make sure you can draw the graphs and label them clearly.
- Explain how heart rate is regulated during physical activity (neural, hormonal and intrinsic control).
- Critically evaluate the impact of different types of exercise on the cardiac system.

Response of the vascular system to physical activity

The venous return mechanism

Venous return is the term used for the return of blood to the right side of the heart through the veins.

At rest, 70% of the total blood volume is contained in the veins. This provides a large reservoir of blood that can be returned rapidly to the heart when needed. The heart can only pump out as much blood as it receives, so cardiac output depends on venous return. A rapid increase in venous return enables a significant increase in stroke volume and, therefore, cardiac output. Veins have a large lumen and offer little resistance to blood flow. By the time blood enters the veins, blood pressure is low. This means that active mechanisms are needed to ensure venous return:

- **Skeletal muscle pump** — when muscles contract and relax they change shape. This change in shape means that the muscles press on the nearby veins, causing a pumping effect and squeezing the blood towards the heart.
- **Respiratory pump** — when muscles contract and relax during inspiration and expiration, pressure changes occur in the thoracic and abdominal cavities. These pressure changes compress the nearby veins and enable blood to return to the heart.

- **Valves** — it is important that blood in the veins flows in only one direction. The presence of valves ensures that this happens. This is because once the blood has passed through a valve, the valve closes to prevent the blood from flowing back.
- **Smooth muscle** — there is a thin layer of smooth muscle in the walls of the veins. This helps to squeeze blood back towards the heart.

In addition, **gravity** assists the flow of blood from body parts above the heart.

Vasomotor control

The **vasomotor centre** in the medulla of the brain controls blood pressure and blood flow. The vasomotor centre is stimulated by:
- chemoreceptors, which detect chemical changes
- baroreceptors, which respond to changes in blood pressure

Blood flow is then redistributed through **vasodilation** and **vasoconstriction**. Vasodilation increases blood flow; vasoconstriction decreases blood flow.

The vascular shunt

During exercise, the working muscles need more oxygen. Vasodilation of the vessels supplying muscles occurs, which increases blood flow and brings in much-needed oxygen. At the same time, vasoconstriction occurs in the arterioles supplying non-essential organs. This redirection of blood flow is called the **vascular shunt**.

Pre-capillary sphincters also aid blood redistribution. These are tiny rings of muscle located at the opening of capillaries. When they contract, the blood flow through the capillary is restricted; when they relax, blood flow is increased. During exercise, the capillary networks supplying skeletal muscle have relaxed pre-capillary sphincters. Therefore, the blood flow to the muscles increases and the tissues are saturated with oxygen.

Transport of oxygen and carbon dioxide in the vascular system

During exercise, when oxygen diffuses into the capillaries in the lungs, 3% dissolves in plasma and 97% combines with haemoglobin in red blood cells, forming oxyhaemoglobin. At the tissues, oxyhaemoglobin dissociates, releasing oxygen. This happens because the partial pressure of oxygen in the muscles is lower than it is in the blood. In the muscle, oxygen is picked up by myoglobin. This has a high affinity for oxygen and acts as an oxygen store. Numerous mitochondria in the skeletal muscles use the oxygen for aerobic respiration, producing the energy needed for muscular contraction.

Carbon dioxide is transported in one of three ways:
- 70% combines with water as hydrogen carbonate (bicarbonate) ions
- 23% combines with haemoglobin to form carbaminohaemoglobin
- 7% dissolves in plasma

Effective transport of oxygen and carbon dioxide helps participation in physical activities

Oxygen plays a major role in energy production. A reduction in the amount of oxygen in the body has a detrimental impact on performance.

An increase in carbon dioxide level results in an increase in blood and tissue acidity. This is detected by chemoreceptors, which stimulate the medulla to increase heart rate and breathing rate so that more carbon dioxide is exhaled and the arterial blood levels of oxygen and carbon dioxide are maintained.

Smoking and oxygen transport

Smoking has a huge impact on the transportation of oxygen. Oxygen combines with haemoglobin and is transported as oxyhaemoglobin. Smokers inhale high levels of carbon monoxide, which has a greater affinity for haemoglobin than oxygen (200–300 times greater). This means that the level of carbon monoxide absorbed in the blood from the lungs increases, while the level of oxygen decreases. Higher levels of carbon monoxide in the blood reduce the amount of oxygen released from the blood to the muscles, which impacts on performance.

Smoke inhalation also increases the resistance of the airways (often through the swelling of mucous membranes) and therefore reduces the amount of oxygen absorbed into the blood.

Blood pressure and blood flow

Blood pressure is the force exerted by the blood against the blood vessel wall and is often referred to as blood flow × resistance.

Ejection of blood by contraction of the ventricles creates a high-pressure pulse of blood (systolic pressure). The lower pressure as the ventricles relax is the diastolic pressure. Blood pressure is measured at the brachial artery (in the upper arm) using a sphygmomanometer. A typical resting value is 120/80 mmHg (millimetres of mercury).

Blood pressure varies in the different blood vessels, depending mainly on the distance of the blood vessel from the heart:

- artery — high and in pulses
- arteriole — not quite as high
- capillary — pressure drops throughout the capillary network
- vein — low

Effects of exercise

During exercise, changes in blood pressure occur. These changes depend on the type and intensity of the exercise. At the start of aerobic exercise, systolic pressure increases while diastolic pressure remains constant. When exercise reaches a steady state and the heart rate plateaus, systolic pressure decreases owing to vasodilation of the arterioles leading to the working muscles. This reduces the resistance exerted by the blood vessels because the lumen is now wider, and lowers mean blood pressure (the average value of systolic and diastolic pressures) to just above resting levels.

During isometric work, diastolic pressure also increases due to an increased resistance in the blood vessels. This is because during isometric work the muscle remains contracted, causing constant compression on the blood vessels, which results in additional resistance to blood flow in the muscles and therefore an increase in pressure.

Hypertension

Hypertension is high blood pressure. It occurs when constricted arterial blood vessels increase the resistance to blood flow. This causes an increase in blood pressure against the vessel walls. The heart then has to work harder to pump the blood through these narrowed arteries. Without medical intervention, damage to the heart and blood vessels is likely, which increases the risk of stroke, heart attack and heart failure.

Control of blood pressure

The vasomotor centre in the medulla oblongata controls blood pressure. Baroreceptors located in the aortic and carotid arteries detect changes in blood pressure and send impulses to the vasomotor centre.

- If blood pressure is high, the vasomotor centre decreases activity of the sympathetic nervous system which causes vasodilation to occur and leads to a reduction in blood pressure.
- If blood pressure is low, the vasomotor centre increases activity of the sympathetic nervous system and vasoconstriction occurs which increases blood pressure.

The effects of a warm-up and a cool-down on the vascular system

Warm-up

A warm-up period helps to prepare the body for exercise.

- The vasomotor centre ensures that vasodilation occurs, so that more blood flows (due to the increase in cardiac output) to the working muscles. This increases the amount of oxygen transported to the working muscles.
- The warm-up increases the temperature of the body and muscles. This results in an increase in the rate of transport of the enzymes necessary for energy systems and muscle contraction.
- The increase in muscle and body temperature decreases blood viscosity. This improves blood flow to the working muscles. The increase in temperature also results in oxygen dissociating from haemoglobin more quickly.
- A warm-up delays the onset of blood lactic acid (OBLA).

Cool-down

Any activity (such as a gentle jog) that keeps the heart rate elevated allows the body to take in extra oxygen, which can reduce recovery time.

- An active cool-down keeps the respiratory and skeletal muscle pumps working. This prevents blood pooling in the veins and maintains venous return.
- The capillaries remain dilated and the muscles are flushed with oxygenated blood. This increases the removal of lactic acid and carbon dioxide.

Impact of physical activity on the vascular system

Regular endurance activity can have an important impact on the vascular system. The arterial walls become more elastic, which means they can cope with higher fluctuations in blood pressure. There is an increase in the number of capillaries surrounding the lungs and the muscles, and a small increase in red blood cells, all of which help to improve oxygen transport.

Research shows that regular aerobic activity can help to prevent vascular diseases such as **arteriosclerosis** and **atherosclerosis**.

- Arteriosclerosis is commonly referred to as 'hardening of the arteries'. It can contribute to strokes and heart attacks. The walls of the arteries thicken, harden and lose their elasticity. Lack of physical activity is a risk factor for this condition.
- Atherosclerosis is a type of arteriosclerosis. It is a common disorder of the arteries in which fat and cholesterol collect along the walls of the arteries. The fat and cholesterol form a hard substance called plaque, which causes the arteries to become narrow and less flexible. This makes it increasingly difficult for the blood to flow.

What the examiner will expect you to be able to do
- Describe the vascular shunt mechanism.
- Explain how venous return is maintained.
- Explain how oxygen and carbon dioxide are transported in the vascular system.
- Explain how the efficient transport of oxygen and carbon dioxide aids participation in physical activity, and how smoking affects the transport of oxygen.
- Critically evaluate the impact of physical activity on the cardiovascular system with reference to an active lifestyle.

Response of the respiratory system to physical activity

The mechanics of breathing

Air moves from areas of high pressure to areas of low pressure. The greater the difference in pressure, the faster air will flow. Changing the volume of the thoracic cavity alters the pressure of air in the lungs. Increasing the volume decreases the pressure, drawing air into the lungs from outside. Reducing the volume increases the pressure and air is forced out of the lungs.

- Inspiration — the volume of the thoracic cavity increases owing to muscular contraction
- Expiration — the volume of the thoracic cavity is reduced

Respiratory muscles

Ventilation phase	Muscles used during breathing at rest	Muscles used during exercise
Inspiration	Diaphragm External intercostals	Diaphragm External intercostals Sternocleidomastoid Pectoralis minor Scalenes
Expiration	Diaphragm and external intercostals relax (passive process)	Abdominals Internal intercostals

Control of ventilation

Breathing is controlled by the nervous system, which automatically increases or decreases the rate, depth and rhythm of breathing. The control of ventilation is summarised in the diagram below.

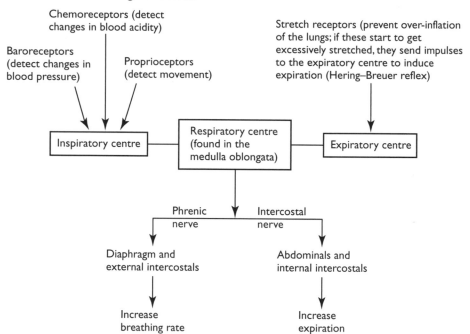

Changes in pulmonary ventilation

Pulmonary ventilation is the technical term for breathing. It is the movement of air into and out of the lungs. At rest we inspire and expire approximately 0.5 litres of air per breath. Changes in pulmonary ventilation occur during exercise. As you would expect, the more demanding the physical activity, the more breathing increases to meet the extra oxygen demand. This is illustrated in the graphs opposite.

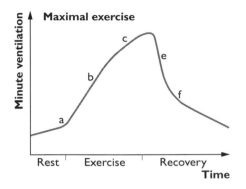

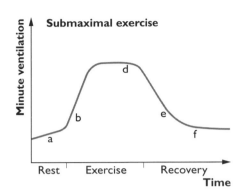

Key to the graphs:
 a = the anticipatory rise
 b = a sharp rise in minute ventilation (the amount of air breathed in or out per minute)
 c = a slower increase
 d = a steady state
 e = a rapid decline in minute ventilation
 f = a slower recovery as the body systems return to resting levels

Gaseous exchange in the lungs

The idea of **partial pressure** is often used when describing gaseous exchange. Oxygen makes up approximately 21% of air, so it exerts a partial pressure. Gases flow from areas of high pressure to areas of low pressure. As oxygen moves from the alveoli to the blood and then to the muscle, its partial pressure in each has to be successively lower.

The partial pressure of oxygen in the alveoli is higher than the partial pressure of oxygen in the blood vessels, so oxygen diffuses into the blood. During exercise, the working muscles use oxygen so the concentration of oxygen in the muscle is lowered and therefore so is its partial pressure. Oxygen diffuses from the blood and combines with myoglobin in the muscle cells.

The difference between any two pressures is referred to as the pressure gradient, and the steeper this gradient, the faster diffusion will be. Oxygen diffuses from the alveoli into the blood, then from the blood to the muscle cells until the pressure is equal.

The movement of carbon dioxide occurs similarly, but in reverse order — from the muscle cells to the blood to the alveoli.

The oxyhaemoglobin dissociation curve

The relationship between oxygen and haemoglobin can be represented by the oxyhaemoglobin dissociation curve on p.30.

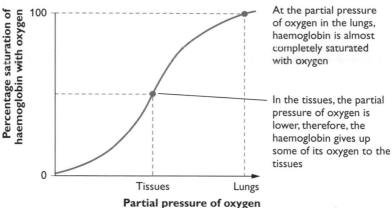

At the partial pressure of oxygen in the lungs, haemoglobin is almost completely saturated with oxygen

In the tissues, the partial pressure of oxygen is lower, therefore, the haemoglobin gives up some of its oxygen to the tissues

During exercise, there is an increased demand for oxygen. The S-shaped curve shifts to the right (Bohr effect). Exercise creates conditions that cause haemoglobin to release some of its oxygen more readily. These conditions are:

- a decrease in the partial pressure of oxygen in the muscle, which increases the oxygen diffusion gradient
- an increase in temperature in the blood and muscle
- an increase in carbon dioxide in the muscle, which increases the carbon dioxide diffusion gradient
- an increase in acidity (lower pH)

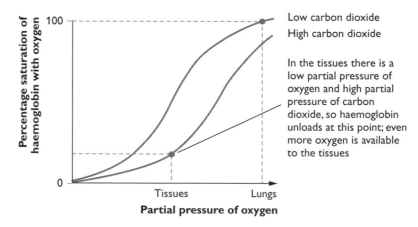

Low carbon dioxide

High carbon dioxide

In the tissues there is a low partial pressure of oxygen and high partial pressure of carbon dioxide, so haemoglobin unloads at this point; even more oxygen is available to the tissues

Effects of altitude training

During exercise, the muscles require more oxygen for aerobic respiration. At high altitude (above 1500 m), there is less air and therefore less oxygen. This lower partial pressure of oxygen has the effect of decreasing the efficiency of respiration. This means the muscles do not receive as much oxygen because the haemoglobin cannot be fully saturated. If the haemoglobin carries less oxygen, there will be a reduction in the amount of oxygen available to the muscles, which will decrease aerobic performance.

With training, the body can adapt to high altitude by increasing the levels of red blood cells and haemoglobin. The advantages of training at high altitude are:
- it increases the number of red blood cells
- it increases the concentration of haemoglobin
- it enhances oxygen transport

Disadvantages of high-altitude training include:
- the expense (cost of flights and accommodation)
- altitude sickness
- initially, training intensity has to be reduced due to the decreased availability of oxygen, which leads to detraining
- benefits are quickly lost on return to sea level

Impact of physical activity

Endurance training improves lung function because the body makes adaptations:
- Small increases in lung volumes occur because the respiratory muscles (the diaphragm and external intercostals) become more efficient.
- The exchange of gases at the alveoli becomes more efficient due to an increase in surface area of the alveoli.
- An increase in the density of the capillaries surrounding the alveoli means that more oxygen can get to the working muscles and waste products such as carbon dioxide are dealt with more efficiently.
- Blood volume increases, mainly due to an increase in blood plasma volume but there is also a slight increase in red blood cells. This leads to an increase in haemoglobin and therefore more oxygen can be taken to the working muscles and more carbon dioxide can be removed.
- Uptake of oxygen by the muscles increases due to an increase in myoglobin content and mitochondrial density in the muscle cells. This leads to an improvement in VO_2max of up to 20%. Having more oxygen available for the working muscles also affects the arterial venous oxygen difference (A-VO_2 diff).

Asthma

Asthma is a chronic disease in which the walls of the airways constrict and become inflamed. During an asthma attack, less air gets into the lungs, which causes wheezing, shortness of breath and chest tightness. Asthma sufferers are often allergic to certain substances, or can react to environmental stimuli such as cold air, warm air, stress or exercise.

Asthma sufferers should be able to take part in most physical activities and regular physical activity can help to manage the disease. For example, aerobic exercise increases lung capacity. Swimming is a good activity because the warm, humid environment is unlikely to trigger asthma symptoms. Scuba diving is the only sport not recommended.

Smoking

Smoking increases the level of carbon monoxide in the lungs. Haemoglobin has a higher affinity for carbon monoxide than it does for oxygen, so the amount of oxygen that diffuses and binds to the haemoglobin is reduced. Smoke inhalation increases the resistance of the airways and therefore reduces the amount of oxygen absorbed into the blood.

Regular aerobic exercise has a beneficial effect in helping individuals to stop smoking. Exercise induces biochemical changes in the body that can increase mental alertness and decrease stress levels. Regular, sustained aerobic exercise increases endorphin levels in the brain, which helps to produce a state of relaxation and wellbeing. Such emotions can help individuals who are trying to stop smoking.

What the examiner will expect you to be able to do
- Describe the mechanics of breathing and the muscles involved, at rest and during exercise.
- Explain how ventilation is controlled.
- Describe the process of gaseous exchange between the alveoli and the blood and between the blood and the tissue cells.
- Explain the effect of altitude on the respiratory system.
- Critically evaluate the impact of exercise on the respiratory system with reference to an active lifestyle.

Acquiring movement skills

Classification of motor skills and abilities

Classification of motor skills

Classification of skills helps teachers and coaches to structure practice in the most efficient way.

A continuum is an imaginary scale between two extremes showing a gradual increase or decrease in characteristic. Continua can be used to classify skills. There are six continua that you need to know.

Muscular involvement
Gross motor skills involve the movement of large muscle groups. Few intricate movements are required. **Fine motor skills** involve precise, intricate movements using small muscle groups.

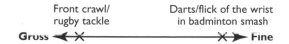

Environmental influence
An **open environment** affects movement skills because the environment is always changing (e.g. the positions of team-mates and opponents). There is much instant

decision making (e.g. in invasion game situations). Skills are usually externally paced and are not predominantly habitual.

In a **closed environment**, skills are unaffected by the environment, which is predictable. They are habitual and follow a precise, well-practised technical model. They are usually self-paced, i.e. the performer has control.

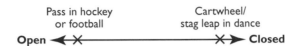

Continuity

Discrete skills have a distinct beginning and end. To be repeated, the skill must be started again.

Serial skills are made up of a number of discrete elements that are combined in a specific order.

Continuous skills have no clear beginning or end. The skill is often cyclic. The end of one skill becomes the beginning of the next.

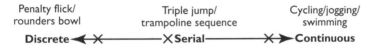

Pacing

The timing and speed of the skill in an **externally paced** movement is determined by the environment (e.g. team-mates and opponents).

In a **self-paced** movement, the performer is in control and determines when the movement starts and the rate at which it proceeds. The skill is usually a closed skill and can therefore become habitual.

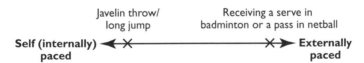

> **Tip** Make sure you do not repeat the question in your answer. For example, if a question asks you to define an externally paced skill, do not write '…a skill where someone else decides the pace of the skill'. Choose words such as 'rate' or 'speed', rather than pace.

Difficulty

Simple skills involve limited information to process and few decisions to make. A small number of subroutines (i.e. parts of a skill) are involved in which speed and timing are not critical. Perception is not used and the use of feedback is not significant.

Complex skills require a lot of decision-making. Many subroutines are involved in which speed and timing are crucial. Perception is required and the use of feedback is important to performance.

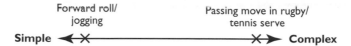

Organisation

Movement skills that are **low in organisation** are easily broken down into subroutines, which can be practised on their own.

Movement skills that are **high in organisation** are hard to break down into subroutines without disrupting the skill and should therefore be practised as a whole. This type of skill is often fast or ballistic.

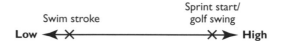

Example

A **tennis serve** is:

- gross, because several of the large muscle groups are used
- closed, because the environment does not change
- discrete, because it has a distinct beginning and end
- self-paced, because the performer controls the speed and timing
- complex, because several decisions have to be made, perception is used and feedback is needed
- low in organisation because it can easily be broken down into subroutines

Applying classification to the organisation and determination of practice

Classifying skills is important for coaches because the classification dictates the type of practice methods that should be used and the way the skill is presented to the learner.

Methods of manipulating skills to facilitate learning and improve performance

Once the classification and organisation of the movement to be taught have been considered, the best method in which to present the skill to the learner must be decided. The best practice method will allow the skill to become grooved or over-learned.

Part practice

Part practice involves breaking down the skill into its subroutines and practising each part until it is flawless. This method works best for skills that are low in organisation and which are easily broken down into subroutines. It is also useful for serial skills, since each element can be practised independently.

Part practice is useful for **cognitive** learners because the focus is on one part of the skill, reducing the possibility of overload and fatigue, especially if the skill is physically demanding. Part practice can also be used effectively for complex or dangerous tasks.

Part practice allows the performer to gradually build confidence, and increases motivation and understanding. However, it is very time consuming and the performer does not develop a 'feel' for the whole skill (kinaesthesis).

Progressive part method
The progressive part method is sometimes called 'chaining'. The first subroutine or part of the skill is practised until it is perfect. The other parts are added sequentially until the whole skill can be performed. For example, the sequence for teaching the triple jump would be:
- practise the hop
- practise the step
- practise the hop and step
- practise the jump
- practise the hop, step and jump

Whole practice
Whole practice is best for skills that are high in organisation and therefore difficult to break down into subroutines. It is good for continuous skills such as cycling and jogging. It is the best method to use for simple, discrete skills where a single action is required, as in a forward roll. If the performer is in the **autonomous** phase of learning, it is best to practise the skill using whole practice. Whenever possible, skills should be taught as a whole, so that the learner develops the correct 'feel' or kinaesthesis of the skill.

Advantages of whole practice include:
- it is less time-consuming because the subroutines do not have to be assembled
- the performer can create a clear mental image of the whole skill, which is easily transferred to 'real' game situations

Disadvantages are:
- there is a danger of information overload — the performer might have too much information to process
- the performer must be physically able to complete the whole skill — it is not the most effective method to use with cognitive performers

Whole–part–whole practice
This method begins with the learner being introduced to the whole skill. One subroutine is then highlighted and practised in isolation, and then integrated back into the whole skill. This allows the performer to develop kinaesthesis *and* to improve weaknesses in the skill. Whole–part–whole practice can be used for cognitive performers and for more experienced performers who are encountering problems. It is also useful for complex skills.

An example is teaching front crawl:

- allow the performer to experience the whole skill
- with the aid of a float, practise the arm action in isolation until it is grooved
- practise the whole skill again, with improved arm action

Definitions and characteristics of abilities

Abilities are:

- innate (genetically determined/inherited)
- enduring (long-lasting)
- the underlying building blocks of skill

Types of abilities

Gross motor abilities involve movements of the major muscles. They are related to physical fitness, and include speed, strength, stamina and suppleness or flexibility. For example, a gymnast uses the gross motor ability of flexibility when performing a backwards walkover, and a basketball player uses explosive strength in a slam-dunk.

Psychomotor abilities involve information processing and decision making and then acting on the decision by beginning the movement response. Perception is a key element. For example, a sprinter has the ability to respond quickly to the starter's pistol in a 100m race (reaction time), or a slip fielder in cricket uses manual dexterity (quick movements of the arm or hand) when catching a ball.

> **What the examiner will expect you to be able to do**
> - Classify skills and more importantly justify your classification with practical examples. Give clear examples at the extremes of the continua — giving an example in the middle may be too vague.
> - Describe the methods of practice and relate them to classification. For example, the progressive part method is used for skills low in organisation. You will also be required to link the methods of practice to the three phases of learning.
> - Critically evaluate the methods of practice, giving advantages and disadvantages of each, and support your answers with practical examples.
> - List the characteristics of abilities (remember that innate, genetic and from parents all mean the same thing and will only be credited once).
> - Define and give examples of gross and psychomotor abilities.

Development of motor skills

Phases of movement skill learning

The psychologists Fitts and Posner (1967) proposed that there are three learning phases or stages that relate directly to the acquisition of motor skills.

The cognitive phase

This is the thinking stage. The key points are as follows:

- The learner engages in mental rehearsal and benefits from observing a demonstration.
- Movements appear uncoordinated and jerky. Many mistakes are made. The performer uses trial and error to find the correct method.
- The performer has to think about the skill: full attention is placed on working out the main components.
- Feedback should be extrinsic and positive, to highlight weaknesses.

Tip Do not confuse the cognitive phase of learning with the cognitive theory of learning.

The associative phase

This is the practice stage. It is the longest phase and some performers never leave this stage. The key points are:

- The performer becomes more proficient and makes fewer mistakes.
- Demonstration remains important and feedback should be positive.
- Mental rehearsal can help learning and develop fluency.
- The performer can begin to focus attention on the finer aspects of the skill.
- Control of the skill is largely through extrinsic feedback (KR).
- The learner begins to use intrinsic or kinaesthetic feedback (including KP) to control the skill.
- Motor programmes develop and are stored in the long-term memory.
- The performer uses closed loop control to manage movement.

The autonomous phase

This is the expert stage, at which the skill can be executed automatically. The key points are as follows:

- The movement is fluent, efficient and habitual.
- The correct response is now associated with the correct 'feeling'.
- Attention can be given to fine detail, tactics and advanced strategies.
- Demonstration and mental rehearsal remain important.
- The expert uses knowledge of performance and intrinsic feedback for self-correction.
- Negative extrinsic feedback from the coach aids error correction and helps in fine tuning.
- The performer uses open-loop level 1 control.

Types of guidance

There are four types of guidance that can be used to help the learning process.

- **Visual guidance** can be in the form of a demonstration, a video, a skill card or a coaching manual. It is best for performers in the cognitive stage of learning as it helps to build a clear mental picture of the skill. The information is easily absorbed by the learner. The coach can modify the display — for example, placing a chalked square on a tennis court for the performer to aim for while practising serves.

- **Verbal guidance** involves telling the learner what to do and it can give technical information. It is more useful for learning open skills that require decision-making and perceptual judgements. It is best used at the autonomous stage of learning and is less relevant to beginners. It can be given during a performance and is often used in conjunction with visual guidance.
- **Manual guidance** involves the coach holding and physically 'shaping' the body to give the learner an idea of how the skill should feel. **Mechanical guidance** makes use of a piece of equipment or a device to aid and shape movement. Both these methods are useful at the cognitive stage of learning, especially for tasks that involve an element of danger. They allow the whole skill to be attempted and build confidence.

Note that manual and mechanical guidance have some drawbacks. For example:
- the performer may come to rely on the support/aid
- incorrect kinaesthesis could develop
- bad habits might be instilled
- the performer might become demotivated by feeling that he/she is not performing the skill without the assistance of the coach/device
- the physical contact or proximity of the coach may make the performer feel uncomfortable

Practice methods and their impact on performance of movement skills

Fixed practice

In fixed practice, the same skill is performed repetitively and the environment does not change. Fixed practice is best for closed skills that need to be well grooved or over-learned (e.g. a vault in gymnastics). Fixed practice can be used because:
- the environment in which a closed skill is performed remains the same
- once perfected, the movement pattern does not change

Varied practice

In varied practice, the environment is continually changing. Therefore, varied practice is best for open skills. An example is changing from partner work, to unopposed practice, to 3 v 2 in rugby. Points about varied practice include the following:
- It improves positional play and passing technique in a realistic game situation.
- Opportunities arise for decision-making and the development of perceptual skills.
- Performers learn to adapt techniques to respond to an ever-changing environment.
- Adaptations are stored and, therefore, the experience (or schema) of the novice performer is expanded.
- It improves selective attention. This is the ability to pick out and focus on relevant parts of the display.

Massed practice

Massed practice is a practice session without breaks. It is used when the task is discrete, closed or simple and when the motivation and ability of the group are high. Key points are that:

- skills are grooved or over-learned, so that they become habitual
- it requires a high level of fitness since the continuous nature of this method can be physically demanding although it can be used to develop fitness in lower level performers

Massed practice might be used by a badminton player attempting to perfect a short serve, or a trampolinist practising a seat drop.

Distributed practice

Distributed practice includes breaks, so the session is divided into short periods. It is used when the task is continuous, dangerous, complex or tiring, or when the ability of the group is low. Distributed practice is more effective than massed practice for learning of motor skills. The rest period is often longer than the physical practice time.

Advantages of distributed practice include:

- the rest interval allows physical recovery, which is useful if the performer is not fit
- feedback and performance analysis can be given
- the rest period can be used for mental rehearsal

Distributed practice may be used by a steeplechaser who runs laps of the track followed by a rest period, during which he/she mentally rehearses the performance, visualising the stride pattern, clearing the barriers and water barrier.

Mental practice

Mental rehearsal involves going over a task in your mind. This creates a clear mental image of the skill. A cognitive performer might picture what the skill should look like — for example, a novice tennis player working out the timing of the subroutines of the serve. More advanced performers might go through strategies or sequences of movements in their mind, either during practice sessions or just before a competitive performance. For example, an expert triple jumper about to take a final jump in a competition might visualise the stages of the jump before actually jumping. The performer can imagine the kinaesthesis of the movement — the muscles used in the performance are stimulated even though no movement occurs.

Mental practice allows the performer to visualise success and to focus on the relevant environmental cues. This helps to reduce anxiety and increase confidence in physical performance.

Studies have shown that mental practice alone is almost as good as physical practice, but physical and mental practice combined (i.e. distributed practice) produced the best results.

Information processing

Stages of information processing

The three main stages of information processing are:

stimulus identification ⟶ response selection ⟶ response programming

- **Stimulus identification** — picking up information from the sporting environment and using perception, for example seeing the shuttle coming towards you and determining its height, speed and direction.
- **Response selection** — having interpreted the information (height, speed and direction of the shuttle), deciding what action is appropriate. In this example, deciding in which direction to move and which limbs to re-position.
- **Response programming** — having decided on a movement, the information is sent via the nervous system to the appropriate muscles, so that the movement can be carried out.

Key processes in information processing

The improvement in performance of a skill can be related to various key processes involved in information processing. In order these are:

display ⟶ sensory input ⟶ perception ⟶ memory ⟶
decision making ⟶ effector mechanism ⟶ feedback

- **Display/input data from the display** — the sporting environment and all the information contained in it. For example, for a rugby player the display includes the ball, team-mates, opponents, pitch markings, posts, referee, linesmen, crowd and the coach.
- **Sensory input** — the senses detect information and receptors are stimulated. The three senses involved are vision, audition (hearing), and **proprioception**. Proprioception is the sense that tells us about the position of our bodies and what our muscles and joints are doing, and to feel objects involved in our performance (e.g. the racket or shuttle). Proprioceptive sense consists of touch, kinaesthesis and equilibrium.

- **Perception** — the process that interprets and makes sense of the information received. It consists of three elements:
  - detection — detecting that the stimulus is present
  - comparison — comparing the stimulus to stimuli present in the long-term memory
  - recognition — matching the stimulus to one found in the long-term memory
- **Selective attention** — the relevant information is filtered away from the irrelevant information. Only the relevant information is acted upon while the irrelevant information is disregarded.
- **Translatory mechanism** — once the information has been interpreted by the perceptual mechanism, the correct response is selected in the form of a motor programme and put into action (Whiting's model only).
- **Effector mechanism** — the motor programme is put into action by sending impulses through the nervous system to the relevant muscles, enabling them to carry out the required movement.
- **Feedback/feedback data** — once the motor programme has been put into action, information about the movement is received. This can be intrinsic (i.e. from within the performer) or extrinsic feedback. This information can be used to assist future performances.

Models of information processing

You need to understand both Whiting's and Welford's models of information processing. The models use slightly different terminology but the key processes are the same.

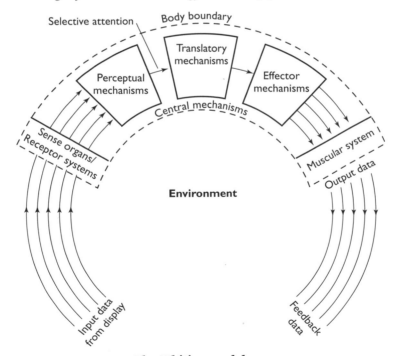

The Whiting model

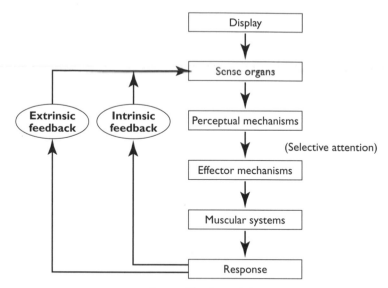

The Welford model

The memory system

The memory system is an integral part of information processing. It stores and retrieves information, makes comparisons with previous movement experiences and selects which motor programme to retrieve in order to produce the movement.

Three components make up the **multi-store model**. You need to understand the features of each.

Short-term sensory store

The features of the short-term sensory store (STSS) are as follows:

- All information is held for a very short time (0.25–1 second).
- Capacity is limitless within the brief time available.
- Selective attention is operational. Relevant stimuli are attended to while irrelevant information is ignored. This is important because it:
  - aids concentration
  - improves reaction time
  - filters out any distractions
  - controls arousal levels
  - reduces the chance of information overload in the STM
- Information is passed to the short-term memory.

Short-term memory

The short-term memory (STM) is known as the **working memory**. The features of STM are as follows:

- It has a limited storage space of 7 ± 2 pieces of information.

- Capacity can be increased by '**chunking**' (see below).
- Information is only stored for up to 30 seconds, unless it is rehearsed or repeated.
- It is responsible for execution of the motor programme.
- Information is encoded and passed to the long-term memory.

Long-term memory

The features of the long-term memory (LTM) are as follows:

- It stores information that has been well-learned and practised.
- Information can be stored permanently.
- It has an unlimited capacity.
- Motor programmes are stored after much practice.

Strategies to improve retention and retrieval

There are a number of strategies that can be applied to help store and remember information.

- **Practice and rehearsal** — repetition 'grooves' a skill and stores the motor programme in the LTM.
- **Linking/association/past experiences** — linking new information with that already stored. For example, a tennis serve can be linked to the fundamental motor skill of an overarm throw (see positive transfer on p 58).
- **Chunking** — small 'chunks' of information can be put together and memorised as one. This expands the capacity of the STM. For example, instead of learning a trampoline sequence as individual movements, the coach could 'chunk' three or four movements together. However, coaches should avoid giving too much information as the STM can easily become overloaded.
- **Enjoyable/interesting/novel experiences** — if learners enjoy an experience, presented to them in a new or distinctive way that they find interesting, they are more likely to remember the information.
- **Meaningful** — if learners understand the relevance of the skill to their performance, they are more likely to remember it.
- **Organisation** — information should be presented in a systematic manner. For example, a tumbling sequence in gymnastics should be learned by practising the individual elements in order.
- **Mental rehearsal/imagery** — if learners can visualise the skill, they are more likely to remember it. This is why demonstrations are important.
- **Reinforcement/rewards** — if learners receive positive feedback or praise after a correct response, they are more likely to remember the information.

Reaction time

Definitions

- **Reaction time** is the time from the stimulus being presented to the performer beginning to respond to it. It is the time from the onset of the stimulus to the onset of the response.

- **Movement time** is the time from the beginning of the movement to the end of the movement. It is the time from the onset of the movement to the completion of the task.
- **Response time** is reaction time plus movement time. It is the time taken from the stimulus being presented to the end of the movement.

For example, in a 100 m sprint:

reaction time: starter's gun goes off ⟶ sprinter pushes on blocks

movement time: sprinter pushing on the blocks ⟶ sprinter crossing the finish line

response time: starter's gun goes off ⟶ sprinter crosses the finish line

Factors affecting reaction time

A number of factors affect reaction time. They include:

- **age** — reaction time increases (slows) with age
- **gender** — generally males have faster reaction times than females
- **stimulus intensity** — if the stimulus is bright (e.g. use of pink balls in cricket) or loud (e.g. a shout), it is easier to detect and reaction time will decrease
- **temperature** — the colder the body, the slower the reaction
- **previous experience** — experience of a skill speeds up reactions
- **anticipation** — predicting a movement correctly can reduce reaction time
- **arousal** — optimum levels of arousal are needed for a quick reaction
- **personality** — extroverts generally react more quickly than introverts
- **drugs and alcohol** — drugs such as anabolic steroids can speed reaction time up but alcohol slows it down
- **limbs** — hands are usually quicker than feet to react, and the preferred side of the body is usually quicker
- **choices** — the more choices we are presented with, the slower we react (see Hick's law below)

Types of reaction time

Simple reaction time is the time taken for a sports performer to react to a single stimulus when there is only one response. Simple reaction time will be short. For example, in a swimming race, the stimulus is the starter signal and the only response is to dive in.

Choice reaction time occurs when there is more than one stimulus and/or more than one response. Choice reaction time will be slower. For example, in football in open play, you may have several team-mates calling for a pass, and several possible responses in terms of who you pass to and what type of pass you use.

Hick's law

Hick's law states that as the number of choices increases, so does the reaction time. In other words, the more choices there are, the slower the reaction time, as illustrated in the graph opposite.

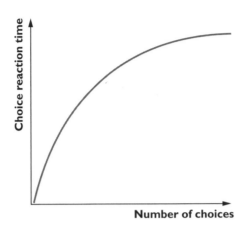

Strategies to improve the response time of a performer

There are a number of ways in which teachers and coaches can try to improve (reduce) the response time of a performer. These include:

- **practice** — the more a stimulus is responded to, the faster the reaction time becomes
- **selective attention** — getting the performer to concentrate on the relevant information and ignore everything else
- **mental rehearsal** — going over responses in the mind ensures that the correct cues are attended to and the appropriate stimuli are responded to
- **experience** — participating in the activity gives insight and awareness of the stimulus being presented
- improve **physical fitness**
- **warm up** — this ensures that the cardiorespiratory, vascular and neuromuscular systems are prepared
- **optimum arousal** — peak levels of arousal ensure fastest response times
- **early cue detection** — analysing the opponent's play (e.g. body/limb position, line-out calls) in order to anticipate what he/she intends to do
- **anticipation** — predicting a movement before it occurs. If a performer anticipates correctly, his/her response time will be very quick and he/she will have more time to perform the skill. However, if the performer anticipates incorrectly, response time can increase greatly.

Psychological refractory period

This is the negative side of anticipation. If we anticipate something incorrectly, then our reactions are slower. If we detect a stimulus and are processing that information when a second stimulus arrives, we cannot attend to the second stimulus until we have finished processing the first. We can only deal with one piece of information at a time (the single-channel hypothesis). This delay in processing information increases reaction time. The delay is called the **psychological refractory period** (PRP).

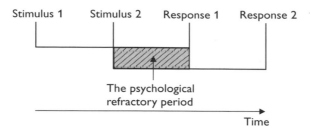

We can use this in sport to slow the opposition down. For example, in rugby you are approaching an opponent with the ball in your hands; you feign a pass to the left. This is the first stimulus and he/she begins to move in that direction. However, you decide to play a dummy and quickly run past without releasing the ball. This is the second stimulus. According to the single channel hypothesis, the opponent has to process the first stimulus of the left pass before the second stimulus can be attended to.

What the examiner will expect you to be able to do
- Describe Welford's and Whiting's models and explain each component using practical examples. Ideally, you should use the same example throughout.
- Describe the multi-store model of memory.
- Describe strategies to improve the storage and retrieval of information. Make sure you can identify and describe the methods.
- Describe the importance of selective attention to the STM — that it filters the relevant information from the irrelevant and without it the STM would overload.
- Define reaction time, movement time and response time using practical examples. The sprint start is the easiest example.
- Demonstrate knowledge and understanding of theories relating to reaction time (PRP, single-channel hypothesis, Hick's law and the role of anticipation).

Motor control of skills

Motor programmes

A motor programme is a set of movements stored in the long-term memory that specifies the components of a skill. It is made up of an **executive motor programme (EMP)**, which is the plan of the whole skill, and **subroutines**, which are the parts or mini skills.

Motor programmes are formed through practice. When the skill becomes grooved or over-learned, the subroutines appear to be performed automatically without thinking. The parts or mini skills flow together smoothly. At this point, the performer is in the autonomous phase of learning. Each time the motor programme is used, it is modified and adjustments are stored in the long-term memory.

Motor programmes have a **hierarchy** of importance. This means the EMP is more important than the subroutines. The subroutines are **sequential** — they are run in a specific order. For example, the diagram below shows the subroutines of a tennis serve, which is low in organisation. The subroutines are performed in sequence to make up the EMP.

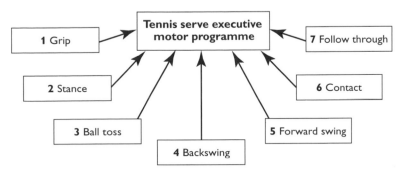

Motor control

Motor control involves manipulation and adjustment of the body during performance to bring about the desired response. The control of motor skills is explained by Adams' **open-loop** and **closed-loop** theories.

Adams suggested that motor control operates on three levels.

Level 1: open-loop control

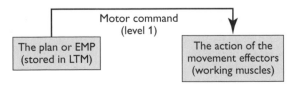

- The EMP is stored in the long-term memory.
- It is triggered by the situation and sent immediately to the working muscles to produce the movement.
- The **memory trace** starts the action.
- Once the EMP has begun, the whole action is produced. The performer cannot change the action.
- No conscious thought is used once the EMP has begun. The action is performed automatically.
- It is used with fast, ballistic, dynamic sporting movements.
- There is no time for feedback owing to the speed at which the movement is produced.

For example, during a sprint start or a golf drive, the performer cannot make any adjustments once the skill has begun. No feedback is used. Alterations can only be made during subsequent performances.

Levels 2 and 3: closed-loop control

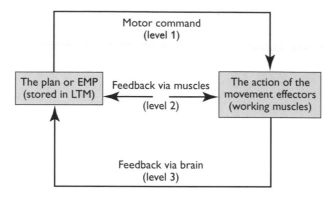

Level 2

- This is a closed-loop system of control where the feedback loop is short.
- The performer makes quick adjustments using intrinsic, kinaesthetic feedback.
- Adjustments are made subconsciously.
- Adjustments are recognised by the brain and stored in the long-term memory for future performance.

For example, a gymnast performing a headstand will make automatic adjustments in body position if he/she begins to lose balance.

Level 3

- This operates on a longer feedback loop because information is relayed to the brain, which processes modifications to performance.
- Conscious thought is used. The performer pays attention to the plan.
- The **perceptual trace** compares the performer's present action with that previously learned and stored in the LTM.
- If the actions match, the performance continues and the motor programme is reinforced.
- If the actions are mismatched, the performer makes the required modifications and a new motor programme is stored.

> **Tip** Candidates often have difficulty with questions about open-loop and closed-loop control. You need to understand each level of control: at level 1 there is no feedback controlling the movement; at level 2 immediate adjustments are made through kinaesthesis; at level 3 conscious thought is used to change the movement. Remember to include as much technical terminology as possible — if you can, discuss the cycle using the terms 'memory trace' and 'perceptual trace'.

Feedback

Feedback is the information received about the skill by the performer during or after the movement. The different types of feedback are summarised in the tables opposite.

Intrinsic feedback	Extrinsic feedback
Comes from within (e.g. proprioceptors and kinaesthesis)	Comes from external sources (e.g. teacher or coach)
Concerns the feel of the movement (e.g. the feeling of balance during a headstand)	Received by sight and hearing and is used to support intrinsic feedback
Important for experienced performers	Important for beginners who have yet to develop the feel of the movement
Novices need to be aware of the need to develop this form of feedback	Can be positive or negative

Positive feedback	Negative feedback
Received when the movement is correct and reinforces the action	Received when the movement is incorrect; prevents the incorrect action being repeated
Can be intrinsic or extrinsic (e.g. positive extrinsic feedback is when a coach praises a novice hurdler for a quick trail leg action)	Can be intrinsic or extrinsic (e.g. negative intrinsic feedback is when a badminton player knows he hit a poor shot because the grip felt wrong)
Used to motivate performers	Reduces the chance of bad habits developing
Essential for beginners	For more advanced performers who may begin to detect and correct their own errors

Knowledge of performance (KP)	Knowledge of results (KR)
Concerns the quality of movement	Concerns the outcome of movement
Technique based: tells you *why* the movement was correct or incorrect	Results based: was the movement successful or unsuccessful?
Can be intrinsic or extrinsic	Extrinsic; can be positive or negative
Important for experienced performers	Important in the early stages of learning and for improving performance

Concurrent (continuous) feedback	Terminal feedback
Received during the movement	Received when the movement is completed or later (e.g. the next training session)
Intrinsic (e.g. proprioceptors and kinaesthesis) or extrinsic (e.g. the coach giving instructions as you perform)	Extrinsic

Feedback is important because:
- performers understand what to do to correct errors
- correct actions are reinforced
- incorrect actions are stopped and bad habits are prevented

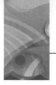

- performers are motivated and their confidence is boosted
- drive reduction is avoided

In order for feedback to be effective, it should be:
- specific to the task in hand
- given in brief, manageable chunks to aid understanding
- compared with previous attempts, to highlight progression
- given immediately
- linked to the performer's personal goals

Schmidt's schema theory

A schema is an accumulation of experiences. Schema theory states that EMPs are stored together in the long-term memory as experiences or relationships with motor programmes. These are known as 'generalised movements' and they allow performers to adapt their skills and **transfer** experiences of one skill to another. This is why some performers seem to be effective in many sports. The performer may take knowledge and skills from one sport, adapt them and transfer them into another situation. The performer's experiences draw together information within the schema from four areas, known as **memory items**.

Type of schema	Functions	Memory items stored each time a movement is performed	Explanation of memory items using a practical example
Recall	Stores information about the movement	(1) Knowledge of initial conditions	Refers to the situation (e.g. whether you have had a similar experience before, in training or a previous game)
	Initiates the movement	(2) Knowledge of response specification	Refers to knowing what to do (e.g. a well-timed pass might be best as it has been successful in similar situations)
Recognition	Controls the movement	(3) Knowledge of sensory consequences (actual feedback)	Refers to kinaesthesis — how much pressure or force to apply (e.g. how hard the ball should be passed)
	Evaluates the movement	(4) Knowledge of outcome	Refers to knowing what the result will be (e.g. the well-timed pass makes it impossible for the defender to make a tackle)

Developing schemata

Coaches can organise practice sessions to enable schemata to develop. For example, they should:
- ensure that practice is varied, to build a range of experiences
- ensure that skills are transferable from training to the game situation

- give feedback to help improve skills
- give praise and positive reinforcement

What the examiner will expect you to be able to do

- Identify a motor programme and its relevant subroutines. These should be given in sequential order to ensure you gain credit.
- Explain the links to open-loop control and the autonomous phase of learning.
- Describe open-loop and closed-loop control and explain the role of each in the performance of motor skills.
- Critically evaluate different types of feedback, with practical examples.
- Explain the relationships of schema theory and motor programmes.
- Identify the four memory items and explain them using a practical example (make sure you use the same example throughout).
- Demonstrate knowledge and understanding of motor programmes linked to your own experience of physical activity.

Learning skills in physical activity

Motivation and arousal

Motivation is the desire to succeed. It is the individual's drive that inspires them to perform well in sport. **Arousal** is the level of somatic or cognitive stimulation needed to prepare an individual to perform (somatic — of the body; cognitive — of the mind).

Extrinsic motivation

Extrinsic motivation is inducement from an outside source. It may be tangible, such as money, trophies or medals, or intangible, such as praise from the coach or crowd. Extrinsic motivation attracts performers to the sport and is therefore a useful strategy for cognitive performers. It raises their confidence and increases participation. However, extrinsic motivation should be used sparingly, especially with young performers, or they may begin to perform for the rewards, and lose the enjoyment and satisfaction gained from performing. For these performers, the withdrawal of extrinsic rewards can lead to total withdrawal from participation.

Intrinsic motivation

Intrinsic motivation comes from within the performer. Participation is for the love of the sport, for self-satisfaction and the pride of achieving one's own goals. Developing health and fitness may be the driving factor. Intrinsic motivation is longer lasting than extrinsic motivation. However, some performers constantly require new challenges to maintain motivation (see drive reduction). Coaches should encourage performers to set personal goals and to generate intrinsic motivation whenever possible.

Drive theory

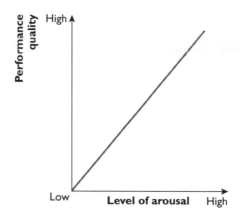

- Drive theory proposes that as arousal increases there is a linear increase in performance quality.
- The performance quality depends on how well the skill has been learned.
- Actions that have been learned are called dominant responses.
- At high levels of arousal, the performer is likely to revert to the dominant response.
- In the associative phase of learning, the dominant response is likely to be incorrect. Therefore, beginners learn best at low levels of arousal.
- In the autonomous phase of learning, the dominant response is likely to be correct. Experts can therefore perform at high levels of arousal.
- If the skill is gross or simple, the dominant response is likely to be correct.
- If the skill is fine or complex, the dominant response is likely to be incorrect.
- Drive theory does not take into account that the performance of elite performers can deteriorate under intense competitive pressure.

Drive reduction theory

Performers have an initial drive or motivation to learn a new skill. Their drive means they will practise the skill until it is mastered or grooved. Once the skill is learned, drive is reduced and motivation levels decrease.

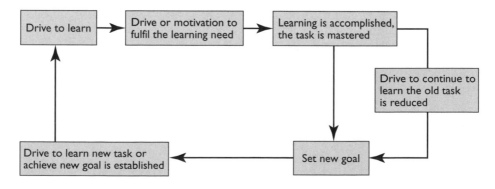

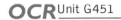

content guidance

Drive reduction theory highlights the importance of maintaining motivation levels, especially with young performers. If they lose their drive or motivation, the performance quality of the skill will decline and they may become disaffected. A new goal or skill must be presented in order to renew their drive.

For example, a young child is determined to learn to ride a bike without stabilisers, and so practises frequently (and develops an active lifestyle). Once he/she can ride the bike properly, practice is unnecessary and the rider becomes disinterested. He/she may begin to lead a sedentary lifestyle. A new goal is required to motivate the child, such as negotiating ramps or completing a course in a certain time. This should provide new drive, improving the chances of the child continuing to lead a balanced and healthy lifestyle.

Inverted U theory

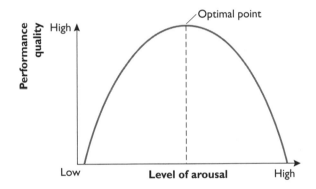

The inverted U theory predicts that as arousal increases, so does performance quality, up to an optimum point at moderate arousal. After the optimum point, if arousal continues to increase, performance quality decreases. Under- and over-arousal are equally detrimental to performance.

If the performer is under-aroused, his/her field of attention will be too broad. The performer is not able to selectively attend to the relevant environmental cues. This may lead to information overload.

At moderate levels of arousal, selective attention is fully operational. The performer can filter the relevant information from the irrelevant, and concentrate on the specific environmental cues required.

If the performer is over-aroused, the field of attention narrows excessively, causing them to miss the relevant environmental cues. In this condition, the performer may be highly agitated or experiencing panic (hypervigilance).

The inverted U theory is more practical because it takes into account the level of performance, the personality type of the performer and the skill classification.

However, it does not account for the dramatic decrease in performance seen by some elite performers once they have exceeded their optimum level of arousal.

Modifications to the inverted U theory

Not all performers operate best at a moderate level of arousal. Some can tolerate only low levels of arousal whereas others may perform at their best at much higher levels, as shown in the diagram below.

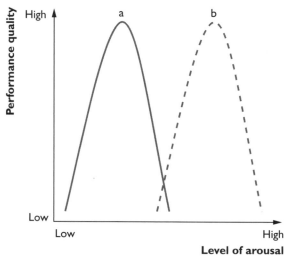

Curve (a) suggests that optimum performance occurs at low levels of arousal. This is generally true for:

- novice performers
- introverts (who naturally have high levels of adrenaline in their bodies)
- fine skills that require a high level of precision and control
- complex skills where decisions have to be made

Curve (b) suggests that optimum performance occurs at higher levels of arousal. This could apply to:

- expert performers
- extroverts (who have low levels of adrenaline and who strive for 'exciting' situations)
- gross skills where precision and control is not needed
- simple skills where few decisions are needed

Catastrophe theory

Catastrophe theory explains the sudden drop in performance experienced by some performers, even at the elite level, when optimum arousal is exceeded. It is the only theory that considers the effects of both cognitive and somatic anxiety.

Catastrophe theory suggests that, as arousal increases, so does performance quality up to an optimum point at moderate arousal — this is similar to the inverted U theory. However, there is then a dramatic decrease in performance as a result of high cognitive anxiety combined with high somatic anxiety. The body and the mind become over-aroused and this causes an immediate and devastating decline in performance.

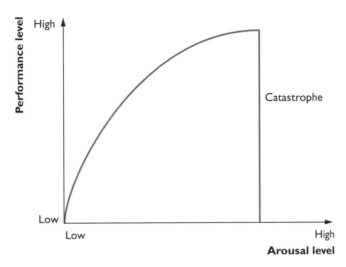

Performing relaxation techniques such as deep-breathing exercises or progressive muscle relaxation can reverse the effects of anxiety. The performer can then continue, provided he/she has reached a level of relaxation below the point of catastrophe.

Motivational strategies

A range of strategies should be used to maintain drive in all performers, or to increase motivation in those who have become disaffected. These strategies may sustain participation and therefore assist in developing a healthy and balanced lifestyle.

For performers in the cognitive stage:
- tangible extrinsic rewards (e.g. certificates, medals, player of the match awards) will attract them initially and should be given periodically
- intangible extrinsic rewards (e.g. praise, positive reinforcement) will increase confidence
- the activity should be fun/enjoyable
- easily achievable tasks should be set, to ensure success
- positive role models or significant others should be identified
- the health and fitness benefits of participation must be highlighted
- varied practice should be used
- responsibility should be assigned collectively — individuals are not to blame for poor performances

For performers in the associative and autonomous stages, the coach should:
- give praise and positive reinforcement

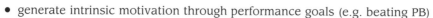

- generate intrinsic motivation through performance goals (e.g. beating PB)
- continually set new, challenging goals, just within reach
- create opportunities to perform with an audience present
- punish lack of motivation
- use peer-group pressure

Theories of learning

Associationist or connectionist theories

Associationist theories depend on linking a stimulus to a response. This link is often called a learning bond or **S–R bond**, where 'S' represents a stimulus (or cue) and 'R' represents the response to the cue. This bond is strengthened by **reinforcement** — the process that causes behaviour to recur.

Operant conditioning

Operant conditioning is a major associationist theory put forward by the psychologist Skinner. It suggests that an S–R bond can be created by manipulating the performer's response. A coach should shape behaviour by:
- allowing the performer to learn by trial and error
- allowing success by giving easy targets
- structuring practice sessions so that the performer will perform the required action — this could include adapting the sporting environment
- reinforcing the correct action by offering praise — if an action is not reinforced it will not be repeated

For example, when teaching a performer to serve in tennis the coach should:
- tell them to 'have a go' using trial and error
- adapt the sporting environment by placing cones in the service box as a target to hit — the cones can be removed later
- move the learner closer to the net to make the task easier to begin with — this ensures success
- when the serve is correct, give the learner praise and positive reinforcement, so that the action will be repeated
- when the serve is incorrect, give negative feedback or punishment to stop the action from being repeated

The learner's response will change — his/her behaviour has been shaped.

Positive reinforcement involves endorsing a performer's action when it is correct, so that the action is repeated. Positive reinforcement can motivate performers to continue participating.

Negative reinforcement involves saying nothing when a correct action is shown, after a period of criticism about a performance.

Punishment is another method of reducing or eliminating undesirable actions. It can take the form of extra training, substitution, fines or bans.

Thorndike's laws

The psychologist Thorndike believed that the most effective way to learn is to form and strengthen a learning bond through the application of reinforcement. Thorndike put forward three laws relating to the application of reinforcement.

- **Law of exercise** — the performer must practise in order to strengthen the S–R bond. If an action is not practised, the bond will weaken.
- **Law of effect** — when a correct action is shown, a 'satisfier' such as praise should be given to strengthen the S–R bond. When an incorrect action is shown, an 'annoyer' such as criticism should be given to weaken the S–R bond.
- **Law of readiness** — an S–R bond can only be created if the performer is mature enough mentally and physically to cope with the demands of the task. For example, the performer must be able to fully understand the components of the task and be physically strong enough to perform the skill.

Cognitive theories

Cognitive psychologists believe that learning occurs by thought processes and developing an understanding or 'insight' into the task, as opposed to the influence of a stimulus and response.

- Gestalt theory is the major cognitive theory.
- A cognitive process is a thinking process.
- Skills should be taught in their entirety, and should not be broken down into subroutines. The learner will gain a greater understanding of the skill and develop kinaesthesis of the whole skill.
- The learner should work out what is required, considering the **intervening variables**.
- Learners should use past experiences of similar situations to help with the current task.
- The learner should use **perception** to make an educated judgement and interpret the information available.

Social learning theory

Bandura's model of observational learning

The psychologist Bandura believed that we learn by watching and copying the actions of 'model' performers, who we respect and admire (**significant others**). Significant others include family members, coaches, teachers, peers or role models in the media. Learners are more likely to copy:

- significant others
- models with similar characteristics, e.g. age, gender
- actions that are successful
- actions that are reinforced

Significant others play a major part in developing healthy, balanced and active lifestyles, especially for young learners. If youngsters look up to healthy role models in their family or in the media, they are more likely to copy the behaviour and lead a healthy lifestyle themselves.

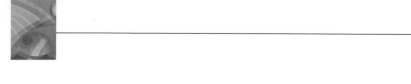

Coaches can use the fact that behaviour is often copied by using strategies to ensure that the learner copies desired behaviour.

- A **demonstration** must be given — behaviour and demonstrations are more likely to be copied if they are consistent, so the demonstration must be accurate.
- The demonstration must grab the learner's **attention**. The coach should ensure that the performer concentrates on the demonstration by making it attractive (perhaps by using a role model) and relevant, and by highlighting the key points.
- The demonstration must be remembered (**retention**). It should be repeated and the information broken down so that it can be recalled more easily. The learner will create a clear mental image through visualisation or mental rehearsal.
- The performer must be physically and mentally able to copy the demonstration (**motor reproduction**).
- The performer must be **motivated** to copy the skill. The coach should offer praise or rewards to increase motivation.
- **Matching performance** — the learner will then match the demonstration.

Transfer of learning

Transfer accounts for the effects that the learning and performance of one skill may have on the learning and performance of another skill. Practically all learning is based on some form of transfer.

You need to know about five types of transfer and to be able to apply them to practical examples:

- **Positive transfer** occurs when one skill facilitates the learning and performance of another. For example, two skills that have similar forms, such as throwing in a rugby union line-out and long passing in American football.
- **Negative transfer** is evident when one skill inhibits the learning and performance of another. For example, a netball player playing basketball may not dribble because he/she transfers the static footwork rule from netball to basketball.
- **Proactive transfer** occurs when a previously learned skill influences the learning and performance of later skills, either positively or negatively. For example, learning to serve in volleyball will help the later learning of a tennis serve.
- **Retroactive transfer** occurs when new skills influence the learning and performance of old skills, either positively or negatively. For example, learning a new golf drive could (negatively) affect your hockey game when you go back to playing hockey because your swing may be too high.
- **Bilateral transfer** is the transfer of learning from one side of the body to the opposite side. An example would be learning to play snooker shots with one hand and then transferring to the other hand.

To ensure positive transfer, the coach should:
- ensure the performer's first skill is grooved
- highlight where transfer can take place
- ensure that the practice environment for both skills is similar

- make practice sessions as close to a game situation as possible
- give praise, reinforcement and rewards when positive transfer takes place

To limit the effects of negative transfer the coach should:
- ensure that the first skill is grooved before the second skill is presented
- highlight the differences in the skills, and therefore where negative transfer may take place
- ensure the performer understands all the components of the skill
- not teach together skills that might seem to lend themselves to transfer but actually don't — for example, a tennis serve and a badminton serve

By transfer of learning from one skill to another, performers build a range of experiences and are able to adapt their motor programmes to suit other situations. An adapted motor programme is called a schema. Some performers appear to have a natural sporting ability that enables them to be proficient in a number of skills and sports. They are in fact transferring skills and using their experiences of other sports to help in the current situation. Schemata are developed through varied practice and should be nurtured in learners as early as possible.

What the examiner will expect you to be able to do
- Define motivation and arousal and distinguish between intrinsic and extrinsic motivation, with practical examples.
- Link motivation and drive reduction with leading a healthy lifestyle. You should explain that a certain level of motivation has to be present in order to maintain performance, and in the case of drive reduction, new challenges should be presented. Therefore performers will continue to participate and lead a more active lifestyle.
- Explain (with the aid of graphs) and give examples for each of the theories of arousal.
- Critically evaluate the theories of motivation. Remember to support your answer with a practical example.
- Discuss the theories of learning and be able to show how a performer learns a skill using each method. Remember to explain how learning from others helps you to lead a healthy, active lifestyle.
- Discuss Thorndike's laws and the strengthening of the S–R bond.
- Describe and give examples of positive and negative reinforcement. Do not confuse negative reinforcement with negative feedback.
- Critically evaluate the theories of learning, supporting your answer with practical examples.
- Describe and give examples of the various types of transfer of learning, with practical examples, particularly for proactive and retroactive transfer.
- Explain the effects of transfer of learning in developing schemata and the importance of variable practice.

Sociocultural studies relating to participation in physical activity

Physical activity

Participation in physical activity

Physical activity can be described as an umbrella term that might include physical and outdoor recreation, physical and outdoor education and sport. For example, an activity such as running could come under the umbrella of physical activity in a number of different ways:

- physical recreation — running or jogging around parks and streets to maintain health and fitness
- outdoor recreation — running up mountains or over fells, incorporating the challenge of the natural environment
- physical education — in school PE lessons or extra-curricular clubs, to improve physical skills
- sport — involving competition against others, with strict rules governing competing and with the aim of winning

Exercise for health

Exercise involves physical exertion for development, training or keeping fit. Your understanding of the term 'exercise' should link to 'the amount and level of physical activity necessary to maintain a healthy lifestyle'. In today's society, people are increasingly sedentary (inactive) and our health is suffering as a result. Obesity and cardiovascular problems are increasing.

Maintaining a healthy, balanced lifestyle

Young people tend to be less active and therefore healthy in today's society for the following reasons:

- safety concerns of playing outside
- fast food diets
- use of transport rather than cycling or walking
- less time for activity during the National Curriculum
- more time spent watching television and playing computer games

Lifelong physical activity/lifetime sport

A government policy has been set up to help people participate in activities that will enrich their lives and their communities. 'Lifelong Learning' will hopefully involve physical activity or sport for many individuals, and will encourage participation in a range of activities that can be continued well into old age, such as swimming, cycling and golf. Such an increase in exercise patterns will have a number of physical, social and mental benefits. It is therefore important to encourage it from an early age.

Schools have begun to offer a broader range of activities as preparation for active leisure, hopefully encouraging lifelong participation. The following strategies are suggested as ways to increase participation in young people and increase the chances of 'lifelong participation':
- provide more appealing PE programmes (e.g. more activity options at Key Stage 4)
- increase school–club links
- set up more outdoor play areas, skateboard parks, outdoor basketball courts and so on
- publicise the availability of facilities and activities (i.e. increase awareness of sporting opportunities)
- subsidise costs of membership to clubs and leisure centres

Possible barriers to regular participation by young people
Young people may be unable to take part in regular physical activity for a number of reasons, including:
- lack of coaching in the activities they are interested in
- lack of equipment and facilities in the local area
- lack of money and the costs of participation
- low skill levels and low self-confidence due to perceived inferiority
- poor PE experience or low status given to PE in their school
- pressure from peer groups can negatively affect participation

Recommendations for a healthy lifestyle
The Health Education Council gives recommendations on physical activity for the general population in relation to frequency, intensity and type of activity. A common recommendation for healthy living is a minimum of five 30-minute sessions of aerobic exercise such as walking, jogging, cycling or swimming per week.

The following recommendations have been made for young people:

'All young people should participate in one hour per day of moderate physical activity; at least twice a week, this hour of physical activity should include activities which help to maintain and enhance muscular strength, flexibility and bone health' (Health Education Authority, 1998).

Physical recreation

Recreation can be defined as the active aspect of leisure. It is entered into voluntarily during free time and people have a choice about which activities they take part in. Any rules are flexible and the emphasis is on taking part as opposed to winning.

Key benefits and functions of physical recreation
People take part in recreational activities to relax, to relieve stress and to improve

their health and fitness. Opportunities arise to meet people and socialise. Society in general benefits from increasing conformity and morality.

Sport

Sport can be defined as highly organised physical activity requiring high levels of prowess, and is usually of a competitive nature. Sport can be identified by a number of key features:

- it involves competitiveness (i.e. a desire to win)
- it is serious, particularly at the elite level
- national governing bodies and officials make up and enforce strict rules and organise leagues and competitions
- it requires a high level of prowess (skill)
- extrinsic rewards are available for success (trophies, medals, money)
- specialist equipment is often used
- time and space restrictions apply
- it involves high levels of endeavour (i.e. maximum effort and commitment to training) to improve performance standards

Key benefits and functions of sport

Sport can serve a number of important functions for individuals:

- keeping a person healthy and fit
- increasing self-esteem and self-confidence as a sense of achievement is experienced
- when joining a sports club, individuals can make friends and socialise

Participation in sport also has a number of important benefits to society:

- less strain on the NHS as people's health and fitness improves
- improved social control as people's free time is spent in a positive manner
- integration of various sections of society through participation of different socio-economic and ethnic minority groups
- financial and employment benefits

Terms associated with sporting ethics

When participating in sport, performers adopt various codes of behaviour, which can be viewed as opposites on a continuum. At one end is **sportsmanship**, which involves treating your opponent with respect and as an equal, playing according to the spirit of fair play and within the rules and etiquette of the game. At the other end is **gamesmanship**, which is the practice of using unfair means to gain an advantage, often against the etiquette of the game but sometimes without actually breaking the letter of the law — for example, wasting time at the end of a game when you are winning, or 'sledging' in cricket when players try to put each other off with verbal comments (as in the infamous Australia versus India test series in January 2008).

Deviant behaviour goes beyond gamesmanship. It involves cheating and going against the accepted rules of an activity. Deliberately fouling or injuring an opponent is regarded as deviant behaviour in sport.

Sportsmanship	Gamesmanship
Kicking the ball out of play when an opponent is injured	Taking a toilet break in cricket
Verbally congratulating the positive performance of an opponent	'Sledging' or using 'verbals' to put opponents off and affect their performance
Trying to stay on your feet and score despite a late tackle	Feigning injury to disrupt an opponent (e.g. taking an injury time-out in tennis)

Physical education

Physical education (PE) can be defined as a formally planned and taught curriculum, designed to increase knowledge and values through physical activity and experience.

Functions and objectives of National Curriculum PE

The aims and objectives of National Curriculum PE can be summarised as:
- physical skills — coordination, body awareness
- health and fitness — physical activity, knowledge of the body, benefits of exercise
- social skills — making friends, improving communication skills
- mental and cognitive skills — decision-making, self-control
- self-esteem — improve self-confidence through success
- leadership — opportunities to lead or captain a group or team
- preparation for active leisure — encouragement and education about the benefits of continuing physical activity into adulthood

Outdoor education

Outdoor and adventurous activities (OAA) should be included as an element of National Curriculum PE. OAA as outdoor education is defined as 'the achievement of educational objectives via guided and direct experiences in the natural environment'.

Functions of OAA as part of NC PE

OAA have many functions, including raising awareness of, and respect for, the natural environment and danger. Risks should be perceived only (i.e. in a pupil's mind) rather than real (actual danger).

Outdoor pursuits such as mountain walking, caving and canoeing can give a personal challenge to individuals, as well as teaching them how to work effectively with each other (teamwork, cooperation). A sense of adventure and excitement and the chance to assume the role of leader are also important elements of the outdoor experience. Communication skills and an awareness of an individual's strengths and weaknesses may develop.

Despite its compulsory status as part of National Curriculum PE, OAA in most schools tend to be of low quality, for example orienteering around the school grounds. The reasons for this include:
- cost
- lack of qualified or motivated staff

- lack of time in lessons
- parents and teachers may be deterred by the inherent risks of OAA

Outdoor recreation

Outdoor recreational activities take place in the natural environment, for example climbing a mountain or canoeing down a fast-flowing river. The challenge of the natural environment is therefore a key feature of OAA. Freedom of choice in leisure time distinguishes outdoor recreation from outdoor education.

Key benefits and functions of outdoor recreation

Individuals choose to participate in outdoor recreational activities for a number of reasons including:
- health and fitness
- stress release, relaxation
- personal challenge, to develop self-esteem
- to develop an appreciation of the natural environment
- to develop cognitive and decision-making skills
- to develop social skills and work as a team
- to develop survival skills

What the examiner will expect you to be able to do
- Demonstrate knowledge and understanding of a range of concepts (sport, physical and outdoor recreation, physical and outdoor education), both in isolation and compared with each other (e.g. characteristics of sport compared with those of physical recreation).
- Apply such knowledge and understanding to a specific activity.
- Define specific terms such as prowess and endeavour; real risk and perceived risk; exercise and lifetime sport; sportsmanship, gamesmanship and deviance.
- Demonstrate knowledge and understanding of recommended targets for physical activity in young people and the barriers that may prevent such targets being reached.

Sport and culture

Sport reflects the culture (customs, sports and pastimes) and society (interacting community) in which it exists.

Sport as a reflection of UK culture

Some traditional sports and festivals have survived over many years. The Highland Games is an example of a surviving multi-sports festival. The key features and reasons for survival are summarised in the diagram opposite.

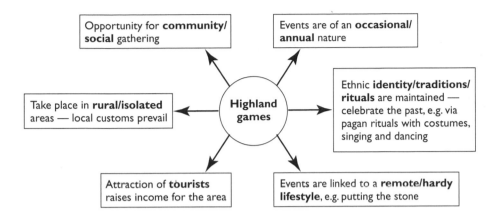

> **Tip** The characteristics of surviving ethnic sports and games are similar to the reasons for their survival, so your answers to questions on either of these should be made from the key points illustrated above (e.g. traditions, social gathering).

The influence of public schools in promoting and organising sport and games

Public schools have a long tradition in Britain, dating back hundreds of years. Games such as rugby and football were played to improve the standard of behaviour among boys attending the schools. The key points are as follows:

- Games were played regularly.
- Boundaries and player numbers were reduced.
- Equipment and facilities became more sophisticated.
- A division of labour was introduced and positional roles emerged.
- Tactics and strategies began to be used.
- A competition structure was devised, initially through the inter-house system, and later among schools.
- Individual school rules gave way to nationally recognised rules (codification).
- Conformity to the rules, fair play and sportsmanship were of key importance — playing honourably was more important than winning.

The move from the traditional 'amateur approach' to a more professional approach

The UK has a decentralised system of sports administration with little government involvement. Voluntary sports clubs at grass-roots level tend to run themselves, with central government providing very little in terms of overall sporting policy, though the provision of lottery money may be linked to achieving certain government targets, such as increased school–club links.

Historically, sport in the UK was organised by volunteers acting as unpaid coaches and unqualified administrators. From small, local, voluntary clubs to national governing bodies (NGBs) and major sports associations, large numbers of unpaid staff were involved in the system, giving it an amateur approach due to lack of expertise in an increasingly commercial environment. An overall policy for sports development was lacking and full-time paid administrators were in short supply. This has led to inconsistency in effectiveness within and among organisations.

In recent years, however, there has been a period of organisational change in sports organisation and administration, which has led to a more business-like approach. Support and interest from the government increased towards the end of the twentieth century and has continued to grow, particularly since the successful 2012 Olympic bid.

The desire for international sporting success has led to increasing numbers of full-time, paid administrators taking up positions in NGBs, particularly in well-funded sports such as football, cricket and rugby. Many NGBs are now appointing performance directors, with sports excellence and the achievement of world titles and gold medals very much in mind as funding allocations are increasingly linked to meeting performance targets.

Sport as a reflection of culture in the USA

The USA is a 'New World' country. It has emerged from a period of colonialism as a relatively young capitalist nation with a population approaching 300 million. Sports played in the USA fall into three categories:
- adaptations — modifications to games already in existence (e.g. American football from rugby)
- adoptions — games taken directly from European cultures (e.g. tennis)
- inventions —new sports designed to suit the 'New World' culture (e.g. basketball)

Sport in the USA is now a multi-million dollar industry, committed to the entertainment market and driven by the profit motive.

The nature of sport in the USA

Sporting events in the USA reflect the US culture, where the win ethic dominates. The mainstream competitive culture has acquired the term 'Lombardianism', after American football coach Vince Lombardi coined the phrase, 'Winning isn't everything — it's the only thing'. Failure in sport is not an option.

Sport in the USA is big business. At all levels it is driven by commercialism. Private and corporate businesses use sport to promote their products, as well as to achieve goodwill. Commercialism of sport starts early, at high-school level. Sport in high school has a high profile and attracts large amounts of sponsorship. Huge crowds are drawn to school sporting events, with pomp and ceremony adding to the entertainment. Those who show the most talent compete for athletic scholarships to go to college or university, where performers receive top-level coaching and support, along with increased pressure to win in a highly competitive environment. College sport is highly commercialised, with funding from television and sponsorship deals. The best college athletes are drafted into professional sport.

Commercialism and sport in American society

Commercialism in American sport is driven by:
- the capitalist society based on material values and a market economy

- commercial enterprise — the USA is seen as a land of opportunity for the individual to make good and achieve the 'rags to riches' ideal
- corporate sponsorship of top sport giving opportunity for advertising
- the impact of the media on promotion and advertising revenue

The American Dream

The American Dream deems that anyone can be a success, irrespective of age, gender or ethnic background, and sport is a particularly useful vehicle for success. Sport can demolish stereotypes and smash through the restrictive glass ceiling of opportunity. Role models on multi-million dollar playing contracts are created, giving others from all sections of society something to aspire to.

Socioeconomic influences on sport in the USA

It is important to understand that US society is driven by capitalism (i.e. the profit motive), which directly influences all that happens in sport from high-school level, through sport at college and on to professional sport. Capitalism allows individuals to accumulate wealth.

The social history of America is reflected by individualism. The USA attracted many early settlers because the land was rich and resources were plentiful. However, before resources can be converted into wealth, they have to be won, often single-handedly. This attitude of every man for himself has steered the USA towards capitalism, with accompanying ideologies such as:
- everyone has the chance to succeed
- freedom is given to all individuals to pursue the wealth and happiness to be gained from capitalism
- happiness is secured through the generation of wealth and achieving the American Dream
- 'win at all costs'/Lombardianism as the mainstream competitive culture

An analysis of American football

American football emerged from the European game of rugby in 1879. Walter Camp, a player and coach of Yale University, instituted the early rules of the game.

The key features of American football are as follows:
- It is a professional sport played to a high standard.
- Huge financial rewards are available for success.
- It has major exposure via the media.
- As a professional sport it gives every player an opportunity to go from rags to riches.
- Massive stadiums accommodate large numbers of spectators, with a family-orientated environment.
- There is support entertainment alongside the sporting event.

American football tends to be of a violent nature. A number of factors can account for this:
- Protective body armour reduces physical inhibition (e.g. the helmet and mask dehumanise performers).

- Head-on contests are confrontational.
- The language is provocative (e.g. 'sack the opponent').
- The culture of the USA— for example, the individual desire for excitement and sensationalism; sports such as American football can be linked to sport as the 'last frontier' (e.g. toughness); the rules and ethos of American football encourage contact, which often leads to violence.
- Media influence — sensationalism and violence in American football sells sport to the public.
- The Lombardian ethic (win at all costs) prevails, with violence seen as necessary for success in many cases.

Sport as a reflection of Australian culture

Australia became independent from the UK in 1901 but evidence of its colonial roots exists in education and sport.

A number of factors influence the Australian national desire to achieve sporting success:
- Settlement and colonialism — the historical influence of Britain.
- Bush culture — the old frontier image of individuality and ruggedness is exhibited through sport.
- Political support — successive governments have recognised the enormous potential of sport to increase Australia's international status and have invested in it. Such investment is seen as reflecting a strong economy and affluence.
- Enlightenment — a healthy lifestyle is important and individuals are keen to take part in sport, particularly in outdoor activities in such a favourable climate. Sport is fashionable and is enjoyed by the majority of the population.
- Unity and nationalism — sport has united a small population in a large land. It has brought different cultural groups together to celebrate sporting success (e.g. at the Olympics).
- Egalitarian society — sport reflects equality of opportunity in society and supports the 'land of the fair go' image.
- Ambition — the desire to be a world sporting power and increase its influence as a nation through sporting success (e.g. in rugby league, rugby union, cricket and Olympic sports).

Analysis of Australian rules football
Factors that have shaped the development of Australian rules football (Aussie rules) into a highly popular sport in Australia include the following:
- It is known as 'the people's game' and is accessible to all; it blends all cultures and celebrates its ethnic appeal (endorsing the egalitarian nature of society).
- Spectators are from all classes and backgrounds, which suits the egalitarian nature of society.
- It reflects the manly image of the bush in the physical, aggressive way it is played.
- It has an image of fair play, which suits Australia and its recognition for the 'best and fairest' (the Brownlow medal is presented to the best and fairest player each year).

- The large open spaces available throughout Australia are reflected in Aussie rules being played on huge cricket ovals with 18-a-side.
- Aussie rules gives opportunities for commercialism through sponsorship and media coverage. It is a good product for television because it allows opportunities for commercial breaks during games. Sport accounts for 15% of television time in Australia and broadcasting games aids various sports, including Aussie rules, by gaining commercial sponsorship. Sky TV is an example of excellent media promotion of the sport and provides extensive coverage. Its recent impacts include:
  – games being played at strategic times throughout the week, to attract the largest television viewer ratings
  – the referee restarting play after goals are scored only when a light on the scoreboard indicates that the television commercial break has ended

What the examiner will expect you to be able to do
- Demonstrate knowledge and understanding of how sport in the UK, the USA and Australia reflects the culture in which it exists.
- Describe the characteristics of ethnic sports and games in the UK, and reasons for their survival, and explain the role of nineteenth-century public schools in promoting and organising sport and games. You also need to be able to describe the organisation and administration of sport and explain how it has changed from the traditional amateur approach to a more professional approach in recent times.
- Understand the key characteristics of the USA as a country and explain the nature of its sport. You should also be able to analyse the key features of American football.
- Similarly, you should also be able to describe the key characteristics of Australia and explain the nature of its sport. You need to be able to analyse the key features of Aussie rules football.

Contemporary sporting issues

Funding of physical activity in the UK

Funding for sport in the UK can be gained from a variety of sources. These can be divided into three main sectors:
- The **public sector** funds sport through central and local government.
- The **private sector** involves companies and businesses sponsoring a team, event or individual in the hope of commercial benefit.
- The **voluntary sector** is where individuals and clubs fund their own training and participation, for example through membership fees. The National Lottery is an important source of funding to local sports clubs and individuals participating in sport in the voluntary sector.

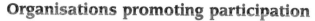

Organisations promoting participation

Sport England

Sport England is a government-funded agency responsible for developing a world-class community sports system. It published a new strategy in June 2008, designed to get more people playing and enjoying sport.

Its key aims are to:
- encourage a million more individuals to do more sport (e.g. via free swimming)
- decrease by 25% the number of 16-year-olds dropping out of sports
- improve talent development in at least 25 sports
- support the 'five hour sport' offer for children and young people (e.g. through the Sports Unlimited initiative and school–club links)

Sport England's strategy is based on the delivery of three clear outcomes:
- **grow** — increasing participation
- **sustain** — maintaining participation
- **excel** — developing talent support systems

Activemark, Sportsmark and Sports Partnership Mark

In 2004, Sport England was involved in discussions with government departments on proposals to develop and reintroduce from 2006 Activemark, Sportsmark and the new Sports Partnership Mark. The key changes were:
- the kitemarks reward delivery of the national PESSCL strategy — this means that only schools within a school sport partnership are eligible
- the kitemarks are awarded annually, through the National School Sport Survey, which all partnership schools take part in

The Youth Sport Trust

The Youth Sport Trust is responsible for developing school sport. It works with a range of partners such as Sport England and Sports Leaders UK. It believes in the power of sport to improve the lives of young people. It considers that all young people should:
- receive an introduction to PE and sport that links to their developmental needs
- experience and enjoy PE and sport as a result of high-quality teaching and coaching, equipment and resources
- be able to progress along a structured pathway of sporting opportunities (e.g. TOP programmes)
- develop a sporting lifestyle as the foundation for lifelong participation

The Youth Sport Trust plays a central role in supporting the government's PESSCL strategy and its key aim of increasing sporting activity among 5–16 year olds. The Youth Sport Trust works with a range of partners, including government agencies, to support the development of specialist sports colleges and school sport partnerships. The Youth Sport Trust also plays an important role in the 'Step into Sport' programme.

UK Ambassadors

Eight hundred young ambassadors are being appointed to spread the Olympic message and to act as role models for other young people.

Talent Matters project

The 'Talent Ladder' website (**www.talentmatters.org**) gives gifted young sports people access to comprehensive information, advice and support. It is a key part of the Youth Sport Trust's Gifted and Talented programme, which is part of the government's overall PESSCL strategy.

School Sport Champion

Dame Kelly Holmes was appointed School Sport Champion to encourage and promote achievement in competitive school sport, which is a key aim of the Youth Sport Trust's work.

UK Sport

UK Sport was established by Royal Charter in 1996. It works in partnership with a number of other organisations, such as NGBs, to develop elite performance standards in the UK. Its mission is '...to work in partnership to lead sport in the UK to world class success'.

In 2006, UK Sport was given full responsibility for high-performance sport in the UK.

Investing in sport: World Class programmes

UK Sport began operating World Class programmes in 1997, with funding from the National Lottery. The aim of these programmes is to support leading Olympic and Paralympic athletes in their quest to win medals and world titles.

A 'no compromise' approach to funding elite sport has been adopted. This means that athletes/sports must reach the targets set, or funding has to be returned. For example, in 2006 the funding for hockey, athletics and basketball was cut as a result of failure to meet the agreed targets. The no compromise approach has led to an increased focus on resources for the most successful performers in the most successful sports.

World Class Events programme

UK Sport coordinates the UK's efforts to bid for and stage major sports events on home soil — for example, the World Cycling Championships in Manchester in March 2008 and London 2012.

Promoting ethically fair, drug-free sport

The UK Sport initiative 'Sporting Conduct' is aimed at improving fair play in the competitive sporting arena. It is also responsible for the implementation and management of the UK's anti-doping policy. In May 2005, UK Sport began its '100% ME' campaign, designed to provide a platform for athletes to celebrate their success as drug-free competitors and to provide positive role models for future generations.

UK Sport and Performance Lifestyle

Performance Lifestyle is designed to help athletes create a unique environment necessary for success. Trained athlete advisors provide advice for competing athletes on how to maximise focus on their sport programme and yet still fulfil other important commitments such as work and family.

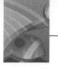

UKSI national network centres

The primary role of each network centre is to assist NGBs and their top performers to reach their targets in terms of world championships and medals. This requires the best coaches, facilities, equipment, sports scientists, medical professionals and various support personnel (e.g. lifestyle advisors). The network centres can also arrange facilities such as warm weather training, acclimatisation, altitude training and winter sports venues.

You can find out more about the work of each institute on the home country websites:

www.sportengland.org.uk

www.sportscotland.org.uk

www.sports-council-wales.co.uk

www.sportscouncil-ni.org.uk

National governing bodies of sport

Some of the ways NGBs try to improve sporting excellence include:
- talent identification schemes
- financial support
- selecting athletes for World Class Performance funding, SportsAid or TASS funding
- giving access to the best facilities and equipment
- training top-level coaches
- providing sports science support (e.g. medical support)
- organising competitions and providing information about them at different levels
- providing lifestyle advice and mentors

Excellence and participation in the UK

The sports development pyramid has four levels. At the bottom is the **foundation** level, which is the first introduction to sport and physical activity for young children. This is often experienced as primary school PE and is sometimes called the 'grass roots' stage.

The second level is **participation**, with an emphasis on fun, socialising and forming friendships in a recreational manner. At school this may be through extra-curricular activities.

Dedicated individuals may reach the **performance** level through regular commitment to improving performance. Such individuals reach county or regional levels of performance and receive specialist coaching to try to improve their standard.

A limited few reach the **excellence** level as elite performers. Such individuals strive to represent their country and are fully committed to their sport.

Sport and mass participation

The idea behind mass participation in sport is that everyone should have the chance to take part as often as they would like and at whatever level they choose. However, reality does not always match this principle of equal opportunities. Target groups identified by Sport England are sections of society that need special attention in order to raise participation levels so that they have an equal sporting opportunity.

Factors limiting participation

Various constraints can limit regular participation in sport:

- **opportunity** — such as time, money and the attitudes of friends and family
- **provision** — the availability of specialist facilities, equipment, coaching and appropriate activities
- **self-esteem** — the self-confidence to take part and the effects of perceptions held by others of an individual or group

Self-esteem is affected by an individual's status in society and can lead to low expectations and under-achievement among the lower social classes, people with disabilities and ethnic minority groups, for example.

Under-representation of women in sport

A variety of reasons can be given to explain the under-representation of women in sport at all levels of the performance pyramid. These include:

- stereotypical myths, e.g. the belief that physical activity could damage fertility, or that women are not aggressive
- less media coverage
- fewer role models and sponsorship opportunities
- lower prize money
- negative effects of school PE programmes, e.g. lack of choice, rules on kit
- lack of time due to work and family commitments
- lack of disposable income
- fewer female coaches and officials

Although the representation of women in sport is still relatively low in relation to their numbers in society, improvements are being made. Reasons for such improvement include:

- greater social acceptance of women having jobs and financial independence
- increased media coverage of women's sport and promotion of positive role models
- stereotypical myths are refuted through education
- more women qualified to coach and officiate in women's (and in some cases men's) sport
- more clubs for women to join and more competitions to enter
- the Women's Sport Foundation (see: **www.wsf.org.uk**) promotes the benefits of participation in exercise, raises the profiles of British sportswomen, and works with other organisations to develop campaigns and policies such as Sports Coach UK and Women into High-Performance Coaching

Race and religion in sport

Barriers to participation and progression to excellence for ethnic minority groups include:

- racism and discrimination
- conflict with religious observances
- a higher value placed on education (less support from family for sports participation)
- racist abuse

- fewer role models (particularly as coaches and managers)
- lower self-esteem and fear of rejection

Possible solutions to racial disadvantage and discrimination include:
- training more ethnic minority sports teachers and coaches, and educating them on the effects of stereotyping
- ensuring there is single-sex provision for Muslim women
- punishing racist abuse more severely
- organising campaigns against racism in sport, e.g. the Kick it Out campaign
- making more provision in PE programmes for different ethnic preferences, e.g. relaxing kit and showering rules to accommodate cultural norms

Under-representation of people with disabilities

Reasons for the low level of participation in sport of people with disabilities include:
- negative self-image, lack of confidence
- lower income levels
- lack of appropriate transport and access into and around facilities
- lack of specialist coaches
- lack of specialist equipment
- fewer competitive opportunities
- low levels of media coverage
- fewer role models
- less funding

Disability Sport England (**www.dse.org.uk**) works to increase participation among people with disabilities. It has a number of important functions, including:
- promoting the benefits of exercise to the disabled
- supporting organisations that provide sport and recreation facilities for the disabled
- increasing awareness and knowledge in society about the capabilities of people with disabilities
- encouraging disabled people to play an active role in the development of their sport

Under-representation of the elderly in sport

The following factors are key causes of the lack of participation by older people (over-60s):
- poor health (e.g. heart problems)
- few specialist coaches catering for the needs of the elderly
- low income levels
- limited choice of appealing activities
- poor media coverage
- few role models

The post-school gap

In 1960, the Wolfenden Report identified a post-school gap of non-participation into which many school leavers fell as they progressed from school/childhood into work/adulthood (i.e. the 16–24 age group). It is therefore important for schoolchildren to have a positive PE experience to ensure that they pursue 'active leisure' on leaving school. This can be achieved through varied and appealing PE programmes, school–club links and by experiencing roles such as coach and official.

Other possible causes of the post-school gap include cost, negative peer pressure and lack of preparation for active leisure. To solve such problems, activities can be subsidised and made more appealing to the youth culture, for example by providing facilities to participate in extreme sports. Schools can link better to leisure centres and introduce students to the activities they provide, for example during Key Stage 4 options programmes.

Current government policies in school PE and sport

The **PE, School Sport and Club Links** (PESSCL) strategy is a national strategy aiming to improve the quality of school PE and sport.

Sports colleges are part of the specialist schools programme, which is run by the Department for Children, Schools and Families. They help to deliver the government's plans for PE and sport by providing high-quality opportunities for young people in their area. Specialist sport colleges:

- serve the local community
- offer links to feeder primary schools, community clubs and UK Sports Institute's network centres
- provide enhanced facilities and top-quality staffing
- receive government grants and lottery funding to improve facilities
- receive increased funding of £100 per student per year

School sport partnerships are groups of schools that receive government funding to come together to enhance sporting opportunities. A partnership team comprises a partnership development manager (PDM), **school sport coordinators** (SSCOs) and primary link teachers (PLTs). Their roles are to enhance opportunities for young people to:

- experience different sports
- access high-quality coaching
- engage in competition

NGBs and whole sport plans

In 2003, Sport England identified 30 priority sports, based on their ability to contribute to Sport England's vision of an active and successful sporting nation. Sport England is working with the NGBs of these sports to develop and implement their whole sport plans (WSP).

Whole sport plans identify how a sport will contribute to Sport England's 'start', 'stay' and 'succeed' objectives from grass roots through to elite level. They enable Sport England to direct funding and resources to NGBs and offer the opportunity to measure how the NGBs are performing.

NGBs are required to open their sport to all sections of society, including those at grass-roots participation levels. Ways of achieving increased participation and sports equity include:

- developing policies linking to specific target groups, e.g. disabled and ethnic minorities

- training more sport-specific coaches to encourage participation
- developing mini-games and modified versions of their sports to encourage participation at all levels of ability, e.g. high-5 netball, short tennis
- making facilities more accessible, affordable and attractive, targeting funds at grass roots levels and inner-city schemes
- improving awareness of sport through publicity, advertising and the use of positive role models

Performance-enhancing products

There are various reasons why performers may be tempted to use drugs, including:
- the potential for improving physical performance and therefore increasing the chance of winning
- pressure from coaches and peers
- the belief that other athletes are taking them
- a 'win at all costs' attitude fostered by the prospect of high rewards (e.g. money and fame)
- a lack of deterrents or a perceived low risk of being caught

It is important to continue the battle against drugs in sport because:
- drugs provide negative role models for youngsters
- they can lead to physical and mental health problems
- drugs are illegal and immoral

In the fight against the continued use of illegal drugs in various sports, possible solutions include:
- stricter and more rigorous random testing
- harsher deterrents and punishments (e.g. lifelong bans)
- the use of positive role models to reinforce the anti-drugs message
- coordinated education programmes for coaches and athletes to highlight the health and moral issues surrounding drugs in sport

Technology in sport

In the increasingly competitive and financially rewarding world of sport, performers and their coaches constantly seek to gain an edge over their rivals. Technological developments can improve performance. For example, a specially designed swimsuit might decrease the drag through the water and improved swimming times as a result, or a pair of football boots might have improvements designed to improve your touch and feel for the ball. 'Hawk-Eye' in tennis might add to your excitement as a spectator as you await the umpire's decision following a player's challenge of a line call. Disabled performers are benefiting from improvements in technology (e.g. Oscar Pistorious and his carbon-fibre blades, which enable him to compete with able-bodied athletes).

Roles of the media

The media have four main roles in relation to sports coverage:

- **Informing** — what's happening in sport (fixtures, results)?
- **Educating** — increasing public knowledge of sport issues such as drugs and hooliganism
- **Entertaining** — helping people to enjoy their leisure time (drama of top-level sport, watching top-class sport on television, reading about their favourite team in the newspaper)
- **Advertising** — helping to generate income for sport, covering sporting events (e.g. the boat race), advertising deals for top performers such as Wayne Rooney

A critical analysis of the relationship between sport and the media

The relationship between sport and the media has both positive and negative outcomes.

Positives	Negatives
Produces positive role models	Sports stars lose their privacy
Brings sport to millioms of people	Audiences may suffer from sporting overload
People may be inspired to participate	Passive viewing and reduced participation may result

The media and sports funding

Television companies pay huge amounts of money to cover sports, and advertisers and sponsors back sport because of the exposure they will get in the media. Many sports have either been adapted to suit the needs of television or have changed their structure to attract television coverage.

There is a direct link between the funding of sport and the media. Media coverage brings sponsors and advertising to sport, which are now essential for many sports to remain viable. Companies sponsor sports mainly as a means of cheap advertising, a way of getting into the public's living room.

This relationship between sport, sponsorship and the media is referred to as sport's 'golden triangle' and it is becoming increasingly essential in the success of sporting events.

Violence in sport

Controlled aggression is a fundamental and necessary part of many sports but uncontrolled aggression can result in injuries and/or penalties.

Performer violence can be defined as 'an aggressive act by an individual outside the rules of sport'. The causes of such violence include:

- a 'win at all costs' attitude
- frustration with officials, opponents, team-mates or the crowd
- local rivalry with the opposition
- receiving verbal or physical abuse
- high rewards of winning
- the physically robust nature of some sports, e.g. ice hockey

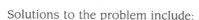

Solutions to the problem include:

- severe penalties, such as bans, fines or 'sin bins'
- the use of video technology by a panel to assess and adjudicate on fair play
- education and emphasis on the ethos of fair play
- a greater number of officials and more authority for the officials

Crowd violence has a number of causes and solutions as outlined in the following table.

Causes	Solutions
Alcohol	Control of alcohol sales
Violent performers	Encourage 'fair play' by performers
Organised gangs	Use of 'police intelligence'
Poor policing/lack of segregation	Improve policing/stewarding
Abusive/racist chants	Use of CCTV to identify troublemakers; harsher punishments

The Olympic Games

Key organisations in the Olympic Movement

The **British Olympic Association** (BOA) develops and protects the ideals of the Olympic Movement throughout Great Britain in line with the Olympic Charter, and supports and leads the best-prepared Great Britain Olympic Team (Team GB) to compete in each summer, winter and youth Olympic Games.

Working with the national governing bodies, the BOA selects Team GB from the best sportsmen and women. Every aspect of Team GB's preparation is planned in detail. This involves organising visits to the host city prior to the Olympic Games and creating an exclusive preparation camp with the best facilities for Team GB to use in the weeks before the Games. This helps Team GB athletes prepare and acclimatise before they settle into the Olympic Village.

The BOA runs programmes to assist athletes throughout their training. These include helping athletes to find jobs that fit around their training and competition, and discounts are provided at national and local sports centres.

For London 2012, the BOA aims to field the largest and most competitive Team GB ever. Its ambition is to finish fourth in the overall medal table.

The BOA's role is defined by three commitments:

- to secure success in the Olympic Games
- to promote, through sport, the Olympic ideals across the 2012 programme
- to deliver a viable London Olympic institute

Hosting the Olympic Games in London will provide a unique opportunity, not just for sport but for the whole of the UK. The basis of the BOA's original dream was to make sure there is a legacy in sport for generations to come.

The **International Olympic Committee** (IOC), based in Lausanne, Switzerland, is the supreme authority of the Olympic Movement. Its aims are to:
- ensure the regular celebration of the Olympic Games
- fight against any form of discrimination affecting the Olympic Movement
- support and encourage the promotion of sporting ethics
- lead the fight against doping in sport
- oppose any political or commercial abuse of sport and athletes
- see that the Olympic Games are held in conditions that demonstrate a responsible concern for environmental issues
- support the International Olympic Academy

Commercialisation of the Olympic Games

The most successful era of corporate sponsorship began in 1984 at the Los Angeles Olympic Games. For the first time, the organising committee for the Games separated sponsors into three categories: official sponsor, official supplier, or official licensee. This allowed the Games organisers and each country's Olympic Committees to generate sponsorship income for the first time. The profit from the LA Games was over $US200 million. In contrast, Canadian taxpayers were paying for the 1976 Montreal Games for decades afterwards.

Sponsorship is now an important source of financial support to the Olympic Movement. Sponsors also provide other support services, such as products, technical support and staff development. Public awareness and support for the Olympic Movement is increased through the promotional activities of the sponsors.

London 2012

Hosting the Olympic Games in London in 2012 will have a number of potential benefits to the UK including:
- improvement in sports facilities in London and the rest of the UK
- urban regeneration and new housing (e.g. a purpose-built Olympic Park will be built for 2012 to include 9000 new homes around the deprived area of Stratford in east London)
- improved transport links and infrastructure
- economic benefits and increased tourism
- raised participation levels
- national pride
- healthier nation, social control
- integration, social inclusion

However, there are some possible negative aspects to hosting the 2012 Olympics:
- relocation of homes and businesses, e.g. compulsory purchase orders will be required to clear land needed for the 2012 Olympic Park
- increased cost to the taxpayers and diversion of funds from other areas of society — council tax rises of around £20 per household are expected
- a legacy of debt if the Games are not commercially successful
- increased security risk, threat of terrorism

- disruption of normal life due to large numbers of tourists
- legacy of unused and expensive facilities

The Olympic Games and nation building

The Olympic Games are often the chosen stage on which communist countries such as China have tried to prove their supremacy in sport and hence show the world that their political system works best. High-profile Olympic sports are therefore chosen for investment by the state, which is often disproportionate in relation to such issues as health and education.

Economic benefits arising from hosting the 2008 Beijing Olympics may also be important for China's nation building, for example increased tourism, a higher level of media attention and advertising, and more investment in industry.

Features of nation building include:
- success creates role models and national pride
- increased tourism and wealth
- appeasement — the nation is kept happy as a result of sporting success
- shop window effect — a feature of sport in communist cultures where success in world events such as the Olympics is highlighted while internal problems are ignored

What the examiners will expect you to be able to do

- Understand the three main ways of funding physical activity in the UK (public, private, voluntary).
- Demonstrate knowledge and understanding of the ways in which a number of different organisations and initiatives promote sporting excellence and mass participation in the UK.
- Explain the terms opportunity, provision and esteem, and how these factors affect participation and achievement in sport, particularly in relation to target groups such as the elderly, the young, people with disabilities, ethnic minorities and women.
- Explain the reasons for the use of drugs in sport and describe the consequences and possible solutions to the problem; explain the impact on performance in sport of modern technological products.
- Explain the roles of the media; critically evaluate the impact of the media on sport, particularly in promoting balanced, active and healthy lifestyles and lifelong involvement in physical activity; explain the relationship between sport, sponsorship and the media (the 'golden triangle').
- Demonstrate knowledge and understanding of violence in sport, both by performers and spectators; describe possible causes and solutions.
- Understand the functions of the IOC and BOA; show understanding of the positive and negative implications of London 2012 for the UK as a host nation; explain how the Olympic Games can be used as a vehicle for nation building, e.g. the 'shop window' effect and use of sport as a political tool in communist countries such as China.

Questions
&
Answers

This section of the guide contains questions that are similar in style to those you can expect to see in the G451 exam. The questions cover all the areas of the specification identified in the Content Guidance section. Your exam paper will have three sections and each of these will have several short questions together with an extended answer question. This extended answer question will be marked by 'levels' and will include assessment of your ability to critically evaluate and your quality of language.

Each question is followed by an average or poor response (Candidate A) and an A-grade response (Candidate B).

You should try to answer these questions yourself, so that you can compare your answers with the candidates' responses. In this way, you should be able to identify your strengths and weaknesses in both subject knowledge and exam technique.

Examiner's comments

All candidate responses are followed by examiner's comments. These are preceded by the icon *e* and indicate where credit is due. In the weaker answers they point out areas for improvement, specific problems and common errors, such as vagueness, irrelevance and misinterpretation of the question.

Question 1
The skeletal and muscular systems

(a) A muscle can perform different types of contraction. The table below shows an example of concentric muscle action.

Action performed	Joint	Active muscle	Type of contraction	Muscle function
Biceps curl (upward phase)	Elbow	Biceps brachii	Concentric	Agonist

Using the biceps curl as an example and the same table headings, analyse another type of muscular contraction that takes place during this movement. (5 marks)

(b) Complete the movement analysis table below by identifying A, B, C, D, E and F.

(6 marks)

Joint	Joint type	Articulating bones	Movement produced	Agonist
Ankle	A:	Talus, tibia and fibula	Plantarflexion	B:
Knee	Hinge	C:	Extension	D:
E:	Ball and socket	Acetabulum and femur	F:	Gluteus maximus

(c) Identify the type of muscle fibre predominantly found in the gastrocnemius muscle of a sprinter. Identify one structural and one functional characteristic of this type of fibre. (3 marks)

Candidates' answers to Question 1

Candidate A

(a)

Action performed	Joint	Active muscle	Type of contraction	Muscle function
Biceps curl	Elbow	Biceps brachii	Eccentric ✓	Antagonist

🖉 The candidate correctly names another type of muscular contraction, for 1 mark. However, because the phase of the action is not specified (i.e. up or down), it is not clear which muscle performs the eccentric contraction, so no further marks can be achieved. In addition, the muscle function is incorrect. Candidate A scores 1 of the 5 marks available.

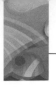

Candidate B

(a)

Action performed	Joint	Active muscle	Type of contraction	Muscle function
Biceps curl (downwards phase) ✓	Elbow ✓	Biceps brachii ✓	Eccentric ✓	Agonist ✓

There is 1 mark available for each correct answer. The candidate has correctly given another type of contraction (eccentric) and named the phase of the action together with the muscle function. This is a top-level answer, scoring all 5 marks.

Candidate A

(b)

Joint	Joint type	Articulating bones	Movement produced	Agonist
Ankle	A: Hinge ✓	Talus, tibia and fibula	Plantarflexion	B: Gastrocnemius ✓
Knee	Hinge	C: Femur, tibia and fibula	Extension	D: Quadriceps
E: Hip ✓	Ball and socket	Acetabulum and femur	F: Flexion	Gluteus maximus

There are a few common errors in Candidate A's answer. The fibula is not part of the knee joint. Including it in the answer renders the whole response incorrect. Quadriceps is not an acceptable answer — you must name a particular quadricep. Always check the movement produced by a muscle. The chances are you know the correct response. Checking through your answers will clarify this. Candidate A scores 3 of the 6 marks available.

Candidate B

(b)

Joint	Joint type	Articulating bones	Movement produced	Agonist
Ankle	A: Hinge ✓	Talus, tibia and fibula	Plantarflexion	B: Gastrocnemius ✓
Knee	Hinge	C: Femur and tibia ✓	Extension	D: Rectus femoris ✓
E: Hip ✓	Ball and socket	Acetabulum and femur	F: Extension ✓	Gluteus maximus

There is 1 mark for each correct answer. This is a top-level answer, scoring all 6 marks.

Candidate A

(c) Fast-twitch fibres. These fibres have a high contraction speed ✓ and fatigue quickly.

Simply stating fast-twitch fibres is not specific enough to score a mark. There are two types of fast-twitch fibre and the candidate should have specified which type is predominantly found in the gastrocnemius muscle of a sprinter. The answer also contains two functional characteristics, rather than the one structural and one functional characteristic required by the question. Therefore, although correct, 'fatigue quickly' cannot score a mark because it is classed as irrelevant. Remember that structure is to do with the make-up of the fibre and that function relates to what it does. Candidate A scores only 1 mark.

Candidate B

(c) Fast glycolytic fibres ✓. These have a large glycogen store ✓ and fatigue quickly ✓.

> ⚡ Sprinting requires maximum effort. The candidate has correctly identified the fibre type as fast glycolytic (Type II b would have been acceptable) and has given one structural and one functional characteristic. Candidate B scores all 3 marks.

■ ■ ■

Question 2

Motion and movement

The effect of a force when applied to a performer can determine the type of motion produced. Using an example from physical education show how you would produce linear motion and angular motion. (4 marks)

Candidates' answers to Question 2

Candidate A

Linear motion is movement in a straight line and angular movement is rotational movement. In tennis you can create topspin and backspin by hitting the ball at the side ✓.

> ⚡ The candidate has explained what linear and angular motion are, instead of saying how they are produced. The first part of the answer is, therefore, irrelevant. Only one example is given, so another mark is lost. If the question asks for examples, make sure you give all of them. Candidate A scores only 1 of the 4 marks available.

Candidate B

Linear motion is when a force is applied through the centre of mass ✓, e.g. a force straight through the centre of a ball makes it move in a straight line in the direction in which the force is applied ✓. Angular motion occurs when a force is applied off-centre ✓, e.g. in a free kick, kicking the ball at the side creates spin or curve ✓.

> ⚡ A correct explanation of how to produce each type of motion is given and there is a relevant example to accompany each answer. Candidate B scores all 4 marks.

■ ■ ■

Question 3
The cardiovascular system

(a) **A 17-year-old cyclist takes part in a maximal effort sprint race. Sketch a graph to show the changes in heart rate before the race, during the race and for 10 minutes after the race.** (4 marks)

(b) **During exercise a performer's heart rate increases. Describe how neural control regulates a performer's heart rate.** (4 marks)

(c) **Explain how blood flow is redistributed to the working muscles.** (3 marks)

Candidates' answers to Question 3

Candidate A
(a)

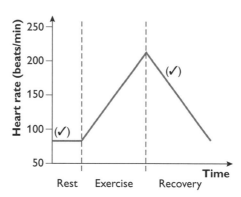

💡 The resting heart rate at the start is correct, for 1 mark, but the candidate does not make it clear that there is an anticipatory increase in rate. The graph then shows a sudden increase in rate but as there is no gradual change, a mark cannot be given. In recovery, 1 mark is awarded for a quick decrease in heart rate, but as this does not become more gradual, another mark is lost. Candidate A scores 2 marks.

Candidate B
(a)

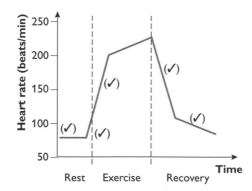

🖉 The candidate correctly identifies resting heart rate as between 40 bpm and 80 bpm. The anticipatory rise just before starting exercise is shown. The graph shows a rapid increase in heart rate up to the accepted range of 140–180 bpm, followed by a more gradual increase between 190 bpm and 220 bpm. During recovery, there is a fast decrease in rate, followed by a more gradual decrease. Candidate B scores all 4 marks.

Candidate A

(b) Baroreceptors, chemoreceptors and proprioceptors detect changes and send an impulse to the brain. This sends an impulse down the sympathetic system ✓ and the SA node is stimulated, causing the heart to beat faster ✓.

🖉 This answer is correct, but because of the lack of detail only 2 of the available 4 marks can be awarded. The candidate should have described what the three types of receptors detect. For example, baroreceptors detect a rise in blood pressure. Using 'brain' is also too vague. The part of the brain (medulla) or the control centre (cardiac) must be specified.

Candidate B

(b) Baroreceptors detect a rise in blood pressure, chemoreceptors detect an increase in acidity ✓. They stimulate the cardiac control centre, which controls heart rate ✓, to send an impulse via the cardiac accelerator nerve ✓. This stimulates the SA node ✓ to increase heart rate.

🖉 This is a comprehensive, detailed answer that gains all 4 marks.

Candidate A

(c) Blood needs to be redistributed to the working muscles because they need more oxygen for energy.

🖉 The candidate has explained *why* blood is redistributed to the working muscles and not *how*. This is a common mistake. Make sure you answer the question. Candidate A fails to score.

Candidate B

(c) An increase in carbon dioxide ✓ is detected by chemoreceptors ✓. An impulse is then sent to the medulla ✓ and vasodilation in the arterioles leading to the working muscles occurs ✓. Vasoconstriction also takes place in the arterioles leading to the non-essential organs ✓.

🖉 The candidate has explained clearly *how* redistribution takes place using the correct terminology, and makes more credit-worthy points than there are marks available. Candidate B scores the full 3 marks.

■ ■ ■

Question 4

Respiration

(a) Describe the mechanism of breathing at rest and explain how this changes during exercise. (5 marks)

(b) Define tidal volume, inspiratory reserve volume and expiratory reserve volume. Describe the changes in these lung volumes that take place during exercise.

(5 marks)

Candidates' answers to Question 4

Candidate A

(a) At rest, to get air into the lungs the volume increases to lower the pressure ✓. This is done by the contraction of the intercostal muscles. When breathing out, these relax ✓. This changes during exercise as more muscles are involved.

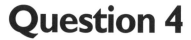 This answer requires more detail. Simply stating 'intercostal muscles' is not sufficient. The candidate should have specified which intercostal muscles are used — external for inspiration and internal for expiration. Expiration at rest is *passive*, which means the muscle relax, and it would have been better if the candidate had used this correct terminology. In this case, however, the candidate was given the benefit of the doubt. During exercise, extra muscles are used; the names of these should have been stated in the answer. Candidate A scores 2 of the 5 marks available.

Candidate B

(a) At rest, the diaphragm and external intercostal muscles ✓ contract, increasing the volume of the thoracic cavity and lowering the pressure, so that air is moved into the lungs ✓. Breathing out is passive ✓. During exercise, this changes because more muscles are used. The extra inspiratory muscles are the sternocleidomastoid, scalenes and pectoralis minor ✓ and the extra expiratory muscles are internal intercostals and the rectus abdominus ✓.

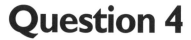 There are 3 marks for describing breathing at rest and 2 marks for the changes during exercise. This is a top-level answer, scoring all 5 marks. However, candidates do not have to give all the extra muscles used during exercise. In this case, one inspiratory and one expiratory muscle used during exercise would have been sufficient.

Candidate A

(b) Tidal volume is the volume of air breathed in and out per breath. Inspiratory reserve volume is the amount of air that can be forcibly inspired after a normal breath ✓ and expiratory reserve volume is the amount of air that can be forcibly expired after a normal breath ✓. During exercise, these all increase.

🗩 Tidal volume is not the volume of air breathed in and out. It is the volume breathed in *or* out per breath. This is a common mistake. The word 'and' changes the whole meaning of the definition. Another common error is to think that during exercise, inspiratory and expiratory reserve volumes increase. Remember these are reserve volumes. If you have to inspire and expire more air while exercising, this means there will be less in reserve! Candidate A scores 2 marks.

Candidate B

(b) Tidal volume is the volume breathed in per breath ✓. Inspiratory reserve volume is the volume of air that can be forcibly inspired after a normal breath ✓. Expiratory reserve volume is the volume of air that can be forcibly exhaled after a normal breath ✓. During exercise, tidal volume increases ✓ and inspiratory and expiratory reserve volumes decrease ✓.

🗩 There are 3 marks available for the definitions (1 mark for each) and 2 marks for the changes that occur during exercise. Make sure you revise all definitions thoroughly and that you know a suitable value for each, as questions sometimes require this additional information. Candidate B scores all 5 marks.

■ ■ ■

Question 5

Gaseous exchange

During prolonged aerobic exercise, a performer requires more oxygen to diffuse into the bloodstream and then to be transported to the working muscles. Explain how gas exchange increases at the lungs to ensure that a greater amount of oxygen is diffused into the blood and then into the muscles, and describe the passage of oxygenated blood as it travels through both the systemic and pulmonary circulatory networks. (10 marks)

Candidates' answers to Question 5

Candidate A

Gas exchange increases at the lungs because the muscles need more oxygen for energy. The oxygen is transported in the haemoglobin to the muscles where it dissociates quickly because of the increase in carbon dioxide ✓. It is then stored in the myoglobin until needed ✓. Oxygen is transported from the lungs to the heart. It goes through the heart and then leaves via the aorta to the body ✓.

🗩 First, the candidate has explained *why* gas exchange increases instead of *how*. Always highlight the words that indicate the requirements of the question — what, why, how, describe, explain etc. The second part of the answer lacks the required detail.

The description of oxygen transport is correct but the candidate fails to mention the chambers, valves and vessels (with the exception of the aorta). Candidate A scores 3 marks out of 10.

Candidate B

Gases move from an area of high pressure to an area of low pressure ✓. During exercise there is an increase in the diffusion gradient ✓. The partial pressure of oxygen is higher in the lungs ✓ and lower in the blood ✓, so oxygen diffuses into the bloodstream ✓. At the muscle there is a lower pO_2 ✓ than in the blood, so oxygen diffuses into the muscle from the haemoglobin to the myoglobin, which has a stronger affinity for oxygen ✓. The oxygen is stored in the myoglobin until it is needed by the mitochondria ✓.

The blood travels from the lungs in the pulmonary vein ✓ where it enters the left atrium ✓. From here it is pumped to the left ventricle and then to the aorta and around the body ✓.

🖉 This candidate gives a simple, logical answer, which makes more credit-worthy points than there are marks available. The candidate has explained how gas exchange increases and described the passage of oxygenated blood. Further marks were available for an explanation of oxyhaemoglobin dissociation and the conditions that speed this process up. Candidate B scores the full 10 marks.

■ ■ ■

Question 6

Classification of motor skills and abilities

(a) Using practical examples, explain the organisation continuum. (4 marks)

(b) Classify and justify the front crawl on the continuity and muscular
involvement continua. (2 marks)

(c) Give two characteristics of ability. (2 marks)

(d) What are gross motor and psychomotor abilities? Use practical
examples to illustrate your answer. (4 marks)

Candidates' answers to Question 6

Candidate A

(a) A skill that has high organisation has lots of rules, a referee and a set pitch. A skill that has low organisation is recreational, with no rules or set playing area.

🖉 Candidates often confuse the organisation continuum with organisation levels in contemporary studies. This answer identifies the extremes of the continuum, but it would be difficult for the examiner to give credit because the explanations are incorrect, and no practical examples are given. Candidate A fails to score.

Candidate B

(a) The organisation continuum is based on how difficult it is to break a skill down into its subroutines. A low organised skill, such as the front crawl ✓, is easy to break down ✓ into its subroutines, e.g. the arm action and the leg action, and practise each part on its own. A highly organised skill, such as a golf swing ✓, is difficult ✓ to break down into its subroutines as it is too fast.

🖉 This is an excellent answer. It explains the continuum and then goes on to describe the extremes of the continuum. Practical examples are given for the extremes and these are very clear, ensuring the examiner will give credit. Candidate B scores the full 4 marks.

Candidate A

(b) Front crawl is continuous ✓ and gross.

🖉 Candidate A has classified the skill correctly but has not justified the reasons for this. It is usual for a sub-maximum to be placed on the answer. Without justification, only 1 mark can be credited.

Candidate B

(b) The front crawl is a continuous skill because it has no clear start and stop ✓. It is a cycle where the end of one stroke is the beginning of the next. It is also a gross skill because it uses a lot of large ✓ muscles in the body.

🖉 This is an excellent answer that addresses both parts of the question. The front crawl is classified and justified for each continuum. You are likely to be asked to justify your classification and the easiest way to do this is to use the word 'because'. Candidate B scores both marks.

Candidate A

(c) Abilities are genetically determined ✓. We get our abilities from our parents. They are stable.

🖉 The question states the number of answers required, so only the first two answers will be marked, in this case 'genetically determined' and 'from our parents'. Although both of these are correct, they are on the same point in the mark scheme and therefore score only 1 mark. The next point is correct but cannot be marked. Candidate B scores 1 mark.

Candidate B

(c) Abilities are the building blocks of skills ✓. Abilities are natural ✓.

🖉 The candidate has answered succinctly and correctly, and scores both marks.

Candidate A

(d) Gross motor ability is using our innate abilities to perform large muscle group movements ✓, for example strength. Psychomotor ability is reaction time.

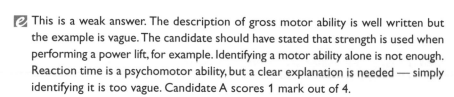

This is a weak answer. The description of gross motor ability is well written but the example is vague. The candidate should have stated that strength is used when performing a power lift, for example. Identifying a motor ability alone is not enough. Reaction time is a psychomotor ability, but a clear explanation is needed — simply identifying it is too vague. Candidate A scores 1 mark out of 4.

Candidate B

(d) Gross motor ability is using your genetically determined abilities to perform large movements ✓. For example, using your stamina in a marathon ✓. Psychomotor ability is about linking the mind with the body. If you have good psychomotor ability, you can process and interpret information quickly ✓, and then send the information to the muscles in order to move. For example, a footballer sees the ball being passed to him/her, judges the speed of the ball, and moves closer towards it in order to receive ✓.

This is a great answer. The candidate has defined gross motor and psychomotor abilities concisely, and has given a clear practical example to support his/her explanations. The candidate has also used the correct technical terminology in the answer. Candidate B scores 4 marks.

■ ■ ■

Question 7

Development of motor skills

Using practical examples, describe the three phases of learning. (6 marks)

Candidates' answers to Question 7

Candidate A

Phase one is the beginners. They are slow and always have to look down and focus on the ball in basketball ✓. Phase two is intermediates. They can look up to pass and make fewer mistakes. Phase three is the experts. They are smooth when passing ✓.

The candidate offers some correct descriptions and examples. However, this 6-mark question requires much more detail and more time should have been given to this relatively straightforward question. Candidate A scores 2 marks.

Candidate B

The first phase of learning is the cognitive phase. Movements are jerky ✓ and the performer makes a lot of mistakes ✓. For example, when dribbling a hockey player might start and stop and lose the ball several times.

In the second stage, the hockey player will start to notice the mistakes and change ✓ body position or grip to rectify them. The performer begins to develop kinaesthesis ✓ and knows how dribbling should feel.

In the final stage the performers are known as autonomous. They are experts. When dribbling they are fluent ✓ and make few mistakes. They can focus on their position on field and where to run to next ✓.

🖉 This candidate shows good exam technique. The three phases of learning are described in turn with an example, and by using the same example throughout he/she clearly distinguishes between the phases. The candidate has not identified the second phase as the associative phase but the question doesn't ask for this and, therefore, full marks can be awarded. Candidate B scores 6 marks.

■ ■ ■

Question 8

Information processing

(a) **What are the functions of feedback?** (3 marks)

(b) **What is selective attention and why is it so important to the short-term memory?** (3 marks)

(c) **Define reaction time, movement time and response time using practical examples.** (3 marks)

(d) **One way of outwitting opponents is by 'selling a dummy.' Explain this in terms of the psychological refractory period.** (5 marks)

Candidates' answers to Question 8

Candidate A
(a) Intrinsic feedback comes from within. Extrinsic feedback comes from an outside source. Knowledge of performance tells you the technical information about your performance.

🖉 This answer is irrelevant. The candidate has described types of feedback rather than the functions of feedback. This is a common mistake when candidates do not read the question properly. This can be avoided by reading the question more than once and highlighting the main words. Candidate A fails to score.

Candidate B
(a) Feedback tells you what you are doing correctly ✓ and detects errors ✓. If a coach tells you that you are doing something correctly, it raises your confidence ✓ and

motivates ✓ you. For example, when you perform a tennis serve correctly, the coach will say, well done, good speed in the serve.

> 🖉 This is an excellent answer. It makes more credit-worthy points than there are marks available and gives a practical example even though one is not asked for. This is good practice. There is some repetition regarding feedback informing you of correct actions — this will not gain further marks but the candidate won't be penalised for doing so. Candidate B scores the full 3 marks,

Candidate A

(b) Selective attention is when a performer blocks out the crowd and focuses on just the ball ✓. It is important to the short-term memory because it can only hold between five and nine items ✓. The short-term memory only lasts between 15 and 30 seconds.

> 🖉 Both parts of the question are addressed. The candidate has not given a clear definition of what selective attention is, but the example would probably gain a 'benefit of the doubt' mark (BOD). Reasons for the importance of selective attention on the short-term memory are given. The points about the amount and length of storage are both correct but are the same points on the mark scheme, and therefore only score 1 mark. Candidate A scores 2 marks out of 3.

Candidate B

(b) Selective attention is filtering the relevant information from the irrelevant ✓. For example, in rugby, the player will focus on the ball and the incoming tackler rather than the rest of the players on the pitch and the spectators. The short-term memory has a limited capacity of five to nine items ✓ and therefore selective attention prevents information overload as it filters away the irrelevant items such as the crowd ✓.

> 🖉 This is a good answer and both parts of the question have been addressed. Selective attention is clearly identified and reinforced with an example. Only 1 mark is available for this part of the question, but this shows the examiner that you have the knowledge and can apply it to a practical situation. The importance of selective attention is discussed clearly, with the aid of a practical example. Candidate B scores the full 3 marks.

Candidate A

(c) Reaction time is the time from when the stimulus is first seen or heard to when you start to move. For example, the time from when the swimmer hears the starter's beep to when he/she dives in ✓. Movement time is the time of the whole movement, e.g. performing the dive. Response time is reaction time plus movement time.

> 🖉 The candidate attempts to address all three parts of the question. Although a little vague, credit would be gained for the answer about reaction time. The answer for movement time repeats the word 'movement' and the example is vague. Response time *is* a combination of reaction and movement time but since no practical example is given, it cannot be credited. Candidate A scores 1 mark out of 3.

Candidate B

(c) Reaction time is the time from the onset of the stimulus to the onset of the response. For example, in the 100 m sprint, this is the time from the starting gun being fired to the sprinter pushing on the blocks ✓. Movement time is the time from the onset of the response to the completion of the task. In the 100 m sprint, this is the time from when the performer pushes on the blocks to crossing the finish line ✓. Response time is the time from the onset of the stimulus to the completion of the task. In the 100 m sprint, this is the time from the starting gun being fired to the sprinter crossing the line ✓.

> 🖉 This answer is succinct and word perfect. The candidate addresses all three parts of the question and gives a clear practical example for each. The sprint start example is usually the easiest to describe. Candidate B scores all 3 marks.

Candidate A

(d) When you 'sell a dummy' this means you go one way then change your mind and go the other. This is the psychological refractory period.

> 🖉 This answer is far too brief for a 5-mark question. It doesn't say what the psychological refractory period is — rather, it just repeats the question. Although it describes a dummy, it does not expand on this in terms of linking the theory to practice. In order to score, the candidate must attempt to do so. More time must be spent on questions with high mark allocation such as these. Candidate A fails to score.

Candidate B

(d) The psychological refractory period occurs when a second stimulus arrives before a previous stimulus has been processed ✓. This is because the brain can only process one item at a time and it causes the performer to freeze. In rugby, the first stimulus from the attacker would be to pretend to pass to the right ✓. The first response from the defender would be to follow ✓ the pass. The attacker would then dummy ✓ and go left, which is the second stimulus. The defender then freezes before changing direction ✓ and going to the left. This is the PRP.

> 🖉 This is an excellent answer. The candidate has read the question and answered it fully, giving a correct practical example as required. Candidate B scores the full 5 marks.

■ ■ ■

Question 9
Motor control of skills

Using a practical example, explain open-loop control. (4 marks)

Candidates' answers to Question 9
Candidate A
Skills are too ballistic or rapid ✓ to get feedback.

  🖉 The candidate has failed to give an example, which automatically restricts the number of marks that the examiner can award. Ballistic and rapid are on the same points on the mark scheme, thus worthy of just 1 mark. The reference to feedback is too vague to gain credit. Candidate A scores 1 of the 4 marks available.

Candidate B
Open-loop control describes how performers control skills that are quick ✓ so that there is no time ✓ for feedback. This could be a skill such as a golf swing ✓. If the performer makes a mistake, there is nothing he/she can do about it. Any changes can only be made next time ✓ round. Once the action has started, the performer doesn't think about it but just performs the skill all the way through.

  🖉 This answer contains little technical language but the examiner will be able to credit the full 4 marks. A clear example is given, as required, and the examiner will award BOD marks with regard to feedback, later adjustments to the skill and conscious attention to the skill. Using more technical language would guarantee marks — don't risk losing marks by being vague.

■ ■ ■

Question 10
Learning skills in physical activity

Using a practical example, describe the inverted U theory of arousal. (4 marks)

Candidates' answers to Question 10
Candidate A
In football, if you are too laid back then you won't perform as well because you are not 'switched on' enough ✓. Similarly, if your coach or team-mates psyche

you up too much, you won't perform as well because you are too aroused ✓ and may fly off the handle.

🖉 The candidate has made an attempt at describing the inverted U theory with the use of a practical example. However, he/she has failed to use any technical language. The examiner would be able to credit 'BOD' marks. The candidate has not explained that best performance is found at moderate arousal levels. Candidate A scores 2 marks.

Candidate B

As arousal increases ✓, do does performance quality ✓ up to an optimum point, which is at moderate arousal levels ✓. Once they have gone past this point, performance will begin to deteriorate as a result of over-arousal. Low and high arousal are equally as bad for the performer. For example, in order to throw a javelin well, an athlete must be at a moderate level of arousal. If they are not aroused enough, they may be too laid back and not throw as far as they could. Equally, it they are aroused too highly, they may begin to panic and again, not throw the javelin as well as they could have done ✓.

🖉 This is an excellent description of the inverted U theory of arousal. The candidate has described the effects at low, moderate and high levels. This type of question will have 3 marks for the description of the inverted U graph, and 1 for the practical example. Without an example, there is a sub-maximum of 2 marks. This candidate has given a clear example which will make it easy for the examiner to award full marks. Remember to read the question properly and always give examples to access the full range of marks available.

■ ■ ■

Question 11
Theories of learning

Compare social learning, operant conditioning and the cognitive theory of learning. (10 marks)

Candidates' answers to Question 11

Candidate A

If you are learning, you are a cognitive performer. This means you are a beginner. Your movements are jerky and slow and you make a lot of mistakes. Your coach has to give you a lot of feedback and you need to watch demonstrations to learn. Bandura says that by watching demonstrations of people we hold in high esteem, known as significant others ✓, we learn from them. We copy their behaviour if it is reinforced ✓. Operant conditioning says that if behaviour is reinforced, it will be repeated ✓. The performer should be allowed to work using trial and error ✓ and the coach should reinforce correct actions through praise ✓.

🖉 The candidate has not read the question properly and has made the common mistake of describing the cognitive phase of learning rather than the cognitive theory of learning. This is irrelevant and is not credit-worthy. The candidate is aware that some links between the parts of the question should be made and has attempted to do so by discussing demonstrations, but not enough detail is given to gain credit. An excellent definition of significant others is given, but this should be supported by practical examples. Bandura's model is not described, but an attempt has been made to describe learning through reinforced behaviour. Finally, the explanation of operant conditioning is better. The candidate has shown some understanding of the method. However, at no point during the answer has the candidate offered a practical example. He/she will not, therefore, achieve higher than level 1.

Candidate B

Social learning theory was suggested by Bandura. He said that performers learn by observing and copying significant others ✓ such as coaches, family members and role models. His model states that in order to learn a skill, the attention of the performer should be focused ✓. This can be done by using a role model ✓ to perform the skill. Then there is retention. This means that the demonstration should be repeated ✓ several times. The performer should be capable ✓ of doing the demonstration — this is motor reproduction. The performer should want to learn ✓ — this is motivation. Then the performer should be able to match the performance.

For example, when learning how to do a netball shot for the first time, the learner can watch an older player in the school who they might look up to ✓. This will grab their attention and make them focused ✓. The player should repeat the shot many times so that the learner gets a clear picture in their mind of how the shot is performed ✓. The learner should also be tall and strong enough ✓ to shoot into the net. If not, the net should be lowered to make it easier for them. Finally, to motivate the learner, lots of positive, extrinsic feedback should be given. This will make them want to continue to practise ✓.

Operant conditioning states that if you reinforce a performer's actions when they do something correctly, they will repeat that action ✓, but if you punish incorrect behaviour it will not be repeated ✓. For example, if a performer is learning to do a football shot and they get the technique correct, the coach should say 'well done' ✓. If they miss the shot or use an incorrect technique like shooting with the wrong part of the foot, the coach could punish them, by giving press ups ✓. In this way, their behaviour is shaped ✓.

These two methods state that skills can be taught in small parts. However, cognitive theory suggests that skills should be kept as a whole ✓ if you want the performer to learn. They should be allowed to work out the best way for themselves and might use their insight ✓ or memory to help them. So, when learning to perform a conversion kick in rugby, the coach should tell the player to attempt it all instead of breaking it down ✓. This is whole practice. The player will work out ✓ how many steps feels comfortable for them in the run up. This means they are working out the intervening variables ✓. They might remember performing a chip pass in football and transfer some of this knowledge when learning the conversion kick, as it is a similar skill ✓. This means they are using their past actions ✓ to help with their new skill. This is a good method for highly organised skills that are difficult to break down and must be learned as a whole.

🖉 The candidate has addressed all three points of the question. The answer illustrates the candidate's knowledge of Bandura's model, and he/she has given a good practical example. To achieve the top level, you must link theory to practical examples at every opportunity. The candidate has also illustrated his/her knowledge of significant others by giving examples. The candidate has sufficient knowledge of operant conditioning and has linked the example of shooting in netball with the theoretical principles. The description of the cognitive theories of learning is described quite well. The candidate has used the example of learning the conversion kick and links this well with a description of the theory. To gain access to the highest marks, you should use specialist technical terms such as 'intervening variables' and 'insight', as this illustrates more comprehensive knowledge. The written communication is fluent and is therefore an examiner would not find it difficult to place this at the top of band 3.

■ ■ ■

Question 12

Physical activity

(a) **PE teachers aim to develop their pupils' knowledge and values. Identify the values and benefits that can be gained from a positive school PE experience.** (4 marks)

(b) **Using practical examples, explain what is meant by gamesmanship.** (3 marks)

(c) **What are the main characteristics of sport?** (5 marks)

Candidates' answers to Question 12

Candidate A
(a) Having a positive PE experience might encourage you to take up sport when you are older ✓. This can improve your health and general wellbeing ✓. Having a good experience can also help encourage your children to participate in sport.

> The first two sentences earn marks as they are linked to the 'preparation for active leisure' and 'improved health' values of PE. The final sentence is vague and confusing. The answer is too brief and lacks a range of different points. Candidate A scores 2 marks.

Candidate B

(a) A positive PE experience can lead to:
- the development of physical skills ✓
- health benefits ✓
- knowledge of the rules of a sport ✓
- help in getting a job or career in sport ✓
- an improvement in self-confidence ✓
- making friends and improving social skills ✓
- knowledge of tactics used in sport

> The first six points are all worth a mark. The final point about tactics is too similar to the earlier point about rules to be credited. This answer is written in an examiner-friendly way with a brief introduction and the key points listed as bullets. More points have been made than there are marks available, to try to ensure full marks are earned. Candidate B scores all 4 marks.

Candidate A

(b) Gamesmanship is swaying the rules in order to win ✓. This may be using drugs.

> The first sentence links to bending the rules without actually breaking them, and scores 1 mark. The attempt at an example is wrong — using drugs is cheating. This answer is too brief. Candidate A scores 1 mark out of 3.

Candidate B

(b) Gamesmanship means using cunning without actually cheating ✓. This may involve distracting an opponent verbally ✓ or wasting time in the latter stages of a game if you are winning ✓.

> The term gamesmanship is explained well. Two relevant practical examples are given. Candidate B scores 3 marks out of 3.

Candidate A

(c) Sport is played professionally at high levels ✓. Professional players such as Wayne Rooney earn a lot of money from playing football for a living. He is a role model. I want to be like him because he plays at a high level for my favourite club. Some of the skills he produces are fantastic, which again makes me want to be like him ✓.

> Although the use of practical examples to illustrate your understanding is encouraged, in this case too much focus on one person has limited the number of marks awarded. Repeating the point about a professional playing for high rewards at a high level means only 1 mark can be gained because the characteristics are so similar. The reference to high skill levels in the final sentence gains a second mark. A variety of points should have been made in answer to this relatively easy question. Candidate A scores only 2 of the 5 available marks.

Candidate B

(c) Sport has a number of characteristics, such as:
- competitiveness and the will to win ✓
- rules enforced ✓
- high fitness demands ✓
- governing bodies (e.g. the FA) ✓
- use of specialist equipment ✓
- officials that make decisions

   🖉 Just enough relevant points are made to gain maximum marks. The final point cannot be awarded a mark because it repeats the point about 'rules enforced'. It would have been a good idea to make one or two more points, in case of vagueness or more repetition. Missing out on maximum marks on relatively easy questions can make a significant difference to the final grade achieved. Unless a specific number is asked for in the question, always make more points than there are marks available. Candidate B scores all 5 marks.

■ ■ ■

Question 13

Sport and culture

(a) **Define each of the following words or phrases:**
   (i) **culture**
   (ii) **ethnic identity**
   (iii) **colonialism**   (3 marks)

(b) **Individual countries approach sport in different ways for different reasons. Identify characteristics of:**
   (i) **sport and the 'American Dream'**
   (ii) **sport as a 'shop window'**   (6 marks)

(c) **Ethnic sports such as the Highland Games continue to survive in the UK today. Give reasons for the survival of such activities.**   (5 marks)

Candidates' answers to Question 13

Candidate A

(a) (i) Culture is where you are brought up.
   (ii) Ethnic identity is your background, which gives you an identity.
   (iii) Colonialism involves colonials going to war and taking over a country.

   🖉 The answer to part (i) is vague and lacks the clarity needed to gain a mark. In part (ii) the candidate repeats a term given in the question (i.e. identity) and fails

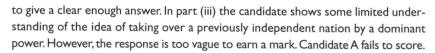

to give a clear enough answer. In part (iii) the candidate shows some limited understanding of the idea of taking over a previously independent nation by a dominant power. However, the response is too vague to earn a mark. Candidate A fails to score.

Candidate B

(a) (i) Culture is how a society lives — for example, its norms, attitudes, customs and traditions ✓.

(ii) Ethnic identity is what makes a person or group unique — for example, race and customs ✓.

(iii) Colonialism is basically empire building. This involves countries such as England taking over other nations and imposing their sports and way of life on them ✓.

There is 1 mark available for each acceptable definition or explanation of the terms asked. There is a tendency among students to leave a gap if unsure of a term. This should be avoided — you have nothing to lose by making an educated guess. Candidate B's answer explains all three terms clearly and correctly and scores all 3 marks. Although not necessary in this case, some concise examples are also given. Such development of an answer is the kind of information you should give if each part of the question were worth 2 marks, rather than 1.

Candidate A

(b) (i) Sport and the American Dream:
- In the USA anyone can achieve success ✓.
- You can go from rags to riches.

(ii) Sport as a shop window:
- Sport is used for political reasons ✓.
- If you can win, it helps politicians.

These answers are too brief and lack the understanding that, hopefully, would have been evident if the candidate had revised this section of the specification more thoroughly. In answer to each question part, a single point is made which is then repeated. Different points are required. Candidate A earns 2 marks.

Candidate B

(b) (i) There are a number of important characteristics of the American Dream, including:
- wanting to win and be the best — the win ethic ✓
- earning lots of money, because sport is seen as a commodity to be bought and sold ✓
- being based on the capitalist principles of a free market ✓
- everyone taking part ✓

(ii) Key characteristics of sport as a shop window include:
- sport being used as a political tool ✓
- competing to try to win for the benefit of your country, not just for yourself ✓
- being based on the capitalist principles of a free market ✓

- the idea that sport can be used to keep the population happy, despite problems, such as lack of food, that may be present ✓

🗨 This shows how a question that is subdivided into two parts should be answered. A similar amount of detail should be given in each part of the answer. This will give a balanced answer with a chance of gaining full marks. Aim to make four or five points in each part of the answer, in case one or more points are vague, irrelevant or repetitive. This is the type of question you should return to at the end of the test if you have time. If you are unsure, include the point, because the principle of positive marking means you cannot lose a mark if a point is wrong. Candidate B gains the maximum 6 marks.

Candidate A

(c) Ethnic sports continue to survive for lots of reasons. An example is the Highland Games, which continues to survive because of tradition ✓. The Highlands want to continue their traditions, which have been going on for centuries.

🗨 The first part of this answer repeats the question, wasting valuable time. A relevant point linking to tradition is made and then repeated. No further relevant points are made. The answer is too brief and lacks the variety of possible reasons required. Candidate A scores just 1 mark.

Candidate B

(c) Ethnic sports continue to exist because of:
- tradition ✓
- religion ✓
- community gatherings ✓
- tourism ✓
- geographical isolation ✓
- a desire to retain ethnic identity ✓

🗨 A bullet-point list is fine here as this question simply asks the candidate to 'give reasons' for survival. This answer is examiner friendly as it sets out six possible answers, which are all relevant, and earns the maximum 5 marks.

■ ■ ■

Question 14

Contemporary sporting issues

(a) **Explain, in relation to the performance pyramid, what is meant by 'sports excellence' and list three different functions of UK Sport that are designed to promote excellence in the UK.** (4 marks)

(b) **Despite harsher penalties and better testing procedures, some sports performers still take performance-enhancing drugs. Identify reasons for this and explain why the fight against drugs in sport must continue.** (6 marks)

(c) **Explain the terms 'opportunity', 'provision' and 'esteem' in relation to mass participation in sport.** (3 marks)

(d) **Discuss the suggestion that hosting the 2012 Olympic Games will benefit the UK.** (5 marks)

(e) **The winning of more medals is affected by many factors. What are the possible effects on elite performance of:**
- **funding (e.g. sponsorship/ National Lottery)**
- **the UKSI (United Kingdom Sports Institute)**
- **the media (e.g. television and newspapers)** (10 marks)

Candidates' answers to Question 14

Candidate A

(a) Excellence is being the best at the elite level of the pyramid ✓. To develop people to the top of the pyramid, UK sport is building more facilities and training more coaches. It also gives out lottery money to help performers develop to the top ✓.

> 🖉 A good, logical start is made, with excellence linked to the word elite in relation to the pyramid. The answer then becomes vague. UK Sport has clear functions in relation to sports excellence in the UK. Unfortunately, many candidates struggle to recall these functions and to write about them in exams. This question asks for a specific number of functions — three — so in this case it is important that the first three functions you state are correct. Candidate A scores 2 marks.

Candidate B

(a) Excellence is identified at the top of the sports pyramid with performers of very high standards ✓.

UK Sport focuses on this excellence level and has a number of functions in relation to it, including:
- the distribution of lottery money to top-level performers through, for example, the World Class Programme ✓

- overseeing the UKSI ✓
- promoting the international status of the UK by attracting major international events to this country ✓

> Candidate B scores full marks. This question requires precise knowledge of key facts, which are often not expressed well by students. This answer is restricted to three key points, as asked. If this is the case in a question, it is advisable to make a quick list of points that you feel are relevant and then decide which points are most likely to earn you marks.

Candidate A

(b) There are a number of reasons why performance-enhancing drugs are still taken, including:
- pressure from the coach ✓
- friends encouraging you to do so
- the win at all costs attitude ✓

The fight against drugs should continue because taking drugs is illegal ✓ and it is cheating. It is dangerous to health ✓ and may have adverse side effects.

> There are elements of good exam technique here. The answer is structured into two separate parts and there is an attempt to make clear, concise points in a bullet-point format, with apparently more points than there are marks available. However, a number of the points are similar and are regarded as 'repeats' of points already made. For example, the first two points are both about pressure. Candidate A scores 4 marks.

Candidate B

(b) There are many reasons for taking drugs, including:
- muscle-building and increasing strength ✓
- losing weight or recovering from injury ✓
- extrinsic rewards and fame on winning ✓
- ineffective testing methods ✓
- poor deterrents and punishments ✓
- because others are taking drugs ✓

Reasons to fight drug taking include that:
- it gives an unfair advantage ✓
- it lowers the status of a sport (e.g. weight-lifting) ✓
- it gives negative role models ✓
- it is cheating ✓

> In a two-part question such as this, there will be a sub-maximum of 3 or 4 marks available. Therefore, a minimum of four points should be made for each part. Candidate B makes ten relevant points, six in the first part and four in the second. The answer is balanced, concise and examiner-friendly as it is clearly structured and the separate points are easily distinguished. The first four points earn the

sub-maximum 4 marks; the maximum of 6 marks is achieved by the two initial points in the second part of the answer.

Candidate A

(c) Opportunity is how much free time ✓ you have to participate.

Provision is how good or widely available sporting facilities are ✓.

Esteem — if you are very quiet, then you may find it hard to fit into a team.

> 🖉 Each answer must be specifically related to the word or phrase given. Candidate A gives correct explanations of 'opportunity' and 'provision'. The final explanation is too vague. Candidate A scores 2 marks.

Candidate B

(c) Opportunity — some sports, for example golf, are too expensive ✓. Can you afford it? ✓

Provision — does your local area provide the facilities ✓ you need?

Esteem — if you are ashamed of your figure or get embarrassed ✓ because you can't play sport, then you might not want to take part.

> 🖉 All three terms are explained well, each scoring the available mark. The last point in relation to 'esteem' is linked to the idea that people lack self-belief. Candidate B scores the maximum 3 marks.

Candidate A

(d) • It will give the UK the chance to be in the media spotlight and showcase the country ✓.
- It will lead to the creation of better sports facilities in the UK ✓.
- Large amounts of money will be generated for the UK.
- It will increase employment opportunities ✓.
- Transportation systems in London will improve ✓.
- Could increase sports participation in the country.

> 🖉 This response answers only one part of the question — the benefits of hosting 2012. This part of the question has been answered very well, with a possible four points made for the 3 marks available as a sub-max. There is some repetition, which should be avoided if possible. The problem is that the issues surrounding hosting the 2012 Olympics are not *discussed* — both sides of the argument are needed. Questions with two parts to them will have a sub-max, which means you need to answer both parts well to score high marks. Candidate A does not do this and scores just 3 out of 5 marks.

Candidate B

(d) Advantages:
- It encourages the nation to unite ✓.
- If successful, our country is seen as strong and successful ✓.
- It gives an opportunity to improve the transport system in London ✓.

Disadvantages:
- It could lead to financial debt ✓.
- Facilities built may be left unused after the Olympics ✓.
- There is a threat of terrorist attack ✓.

🖉 This is an excellent, 'examiner friendly' answer, which clearly answers both parts of the question in the relevant, succinct manner necessary to earn full marks.

Candidate A

(e) Funding increases the provision of specialist facilities where the elite can train ✓. It also helps them buy essential specialist equipment ✓. If they want to go warm-weather training in the winter, lottery money or a sponsor can help pay for this ✓.

The UKSI provides funding for elite performers, which helps cover the cost of travel, coaches, and competition entry fees. Each centre has a specialist sport, such as the Manchester Velodrome for cycling.

The media can have both positive and negative effects on elite performers. Role models are presented to young people who inspire them ✓. The media promote majority sports, such as football, which gets lots of coverage, while minority sports, such as netball, are overshadowed ✓. Media coverage can also promote bad role models and encourage drug taking to become an elite performer.

🖉 The funding answer is good as three relevant points are made, scoring 1 mark each. In this kind of high-mark question, more points could perhaps have been made, supplying more detail and illustrating a wider understanding of the issues involved. The answer referring to the effects of the media is adequate, but repetition of the point about role models (positive and negative) limits the marks. It would have been better to make a different relevant point. The answer referring to the effects of the UKSI is full of incorrect and irrelevant material. To gain high marks in this type of 'banded' question, it is essential to give detailed, correct answers to each part of the question. This is a 'level 2' answer, scoring 5 out of 10 marks.

Candidate B

(e) Funding can help athletes devote themselves full-time to a sport ✓. It helps them to be able to afford the best equipment ✓ and train in the best facilities ✓ with the best coaches ✓ (e.g. Sport England's World Class Programme) ✓.

The UKSI offers top-level performers the chance to work with top-level coaches ✓ in the best facilities ✓, alongside performers at a similar high level who will inspire better performance ✓. Sports scientists are available to analyse and develop performers ✓. In addition, medical support and dieticians are there to help top-level performers keep fit and healthy ✓.

The media can affect top performers because having a great deal of coverage can influence sponsorship opportunities ✓. More people are encouraged to take up a sport and work towards excellence if it gets a lot of media coverage ✓. The media

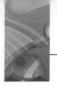

can encourage top performers to do their best and hype up a team or individual. This can either work for or against them — it worked for the rugby World Cup winning England team ✓. Creation of positive role models, such as Kelly Holmes, encourages people to aspire to be like them ✓.

This is an excellent top-band (i.e. 7–10 marks) answer. The candidate gives balanced and detailed answers to all three parts of the question. The inclusion of some practical examples shows clear understanding of the requirements of the question. Candidate B scores full marks.

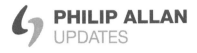
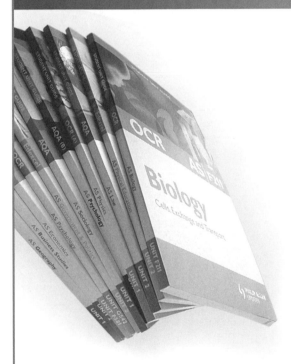

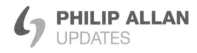
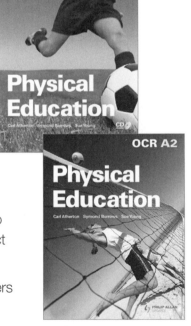